Speaking out

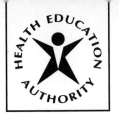

Speaking out

Ros Martin
and
Chrissie Whitehead

Speaking Out first published 1994

© Health Education Authority, 1994

The material in this publication is copyright. The photocopiable originals may be copied for one-time use as instructional material by facilitators, but they may not be copied in unlimited quantities, kept on behalf of others, passed on or sold to third parties, or stored for future use in a retrieval system. If you wish to use the material in any way other than that specified you must apply in writing to the publishers.

Health Education Authority
Hamilton House
Mabledon Place
London WC1H 9TX

ISBN 1 85448 463 X

Typeset by DP Photosetting, Aylesbury, Bucks
Printed by The Cromwell Press, Melksham, Wiltshire

Contents

The Health Education Authority is grateful to the following for permission to reproduce or adapt copyright material

Learning Development Aids for evaluation example 2, 'Field of words', adapted from Tricia Szirom and Sue Dyson *Greater expectations* (1986).

Sheila Kitzinger for handout 6G, 'Assertiveness ladder', adapted from *Woman's experience of sex* (Penguin, 1983).

Impact Publishers Inc. (PO Box 1094, San Luis Obispo, CA 93406) for handout 13D, 'What is assertiveness?', adapted from Robert E Alberti and Michael L Emmons *Your perfect right: a guide to assertive living* (1990).

London Black Women's Health Action Project for handout 14B, 'Female circumcision', from Shamis D-Ashur *Silent tears* (1989).

Many of the materials in *Speaking out* were developed during the Assertiveness and Women's Health Education Project. Every effort has been made to identify materials from other sources.

Acknowledgements

This handbook would not have come about had it not been for the involvement, contributions and encouragement of the following women.

Project facilitators

Bradford: Carolyn Barclay
Bristol: Cathy Benjamin
Cambridge: Franc Johnson
Derbyshire: Charlie Gordon
Exeter: Madie Parkinson
Harlow, Essex: Hilary Durbin
Liverpool/Wirral: Edie Baker, Teresa Roza, Liz Hall
London: Melanie Khan
Midlands: Carole Harte, Lynda Key, Sue Kingswell, Val Gayter
Northamptonshire: Liz Kinross
Poole, Dorset: Maria Boniface
Radlett, Hertfordshire: Michelle McCarthy
Sheffield: Briony Broome, Marget Johnson
Suffolk: Irene Glynn, Suzanne Pearson

Women involved in development work with black and minority ethnic women

Sheffield: Gill Dennis, Carol Jones, Davinder Kaur, Shirley
    Lanahan, Mrs Mohamed, Rubina Rizvi, Esther Wu
London: Maria Boniface, Jacky Downer, Fatuma Hassan,
    Milliee Hill, Amina Ibrahim, Aisha Khan, Melanie Khan,
    Deborah Whall-Roberts

Mary Tidyman, Project Officer, Health Education Authority.
Lee Adams, Project Manager, Director of Health Promotion,
    Sheffield Health Authority.

Marie Goldsmith and Hannah Cinamon, Projects Officers, HIV, AIDS and Sexual Health Programme, HEA.

Isha McKenzie-Mavinga, External Supervisor.

Judy Citron, Evaluator.

Lesley Pattenson, Project Officer at the HEA for the first year of the Project.

Jan Mojsa, Abiola Ogunsola, Dawna King and Junne Baron for facilitating various training events.

Alex Zingas and Michelle Lazurus for their valuable feedback, Margot Jackson for the artwork on the draft materials.

Cherry Eales for her work in setting up the library for the Project.

Jasbar Johal for compiling a dynamic resource list for the draft materials.

All the women who participated in the groups set up as part of the Project's work, or who took part in the Project conference.

All the women who piloted the draft materials.

Foreword

In 1989 the Health Education Authority (HEA) commissioned a study to identify resources and training in assertiveness and women's health education. It found that:

- although women were taking part in work on assertiveness and health in a variety of settings (within health centres, community centres, adult education, etc.), there was very little support and encouragement for women to explore and develop this area of work;

- there were very few resource materials available specifically linking assertiveness and women's health;

- certain groups of women were often marginalised in terms of resources and training.

This information, coupled with the growing recognition that health promotion and health care can be considerably enhanced by encouraging women to support each other and to assert themselves, prompted the HEA to set up the two-year Assertiveness and Women's Health Education Project.

The Project began in January 1990 and worked within different women's communities – often with groups of women whose voices are frequently ignored. The Project aimed firstly to make assertiveness and health work more accessible to all women, and secondly to explore women's physical, emotional and sexual health while building on existing experiences, needs and interests.

One of the outcomes of the Project was the production of this handbook, which involved:

- producing resource materials on assertiveness and health with women already working on the subject with women in the community;

- running residential workshops for these women, to explore the links between assertiveness, health and sexual health;

- organising a national conference dealing with these issues in relation to particular groups of women;

- running a study day on assertiveness and sexual health for black and minority ethnic women;

- facilitating a group and a network for black and minority ethnic women to produce relevant materials based on their understanding of assertiveness, health, well-being and group work in their communities.

This process has enabled us to gather materials from the work that different communities are already doing. These materials have been piloted among women from a range of backgrounds and with a range of experiences.

We hope that *Speaking out* will be a resource that encourages and support your work on health and assertiveness. We hope it will help both facilitators and participants to discover their own assertive and healthy selves.

Introduction

Why assertiveness and health?

Women who join a group on assertiveness may not be aware of the role of assertiveness in their lives, but they have all already used their ability to be assertive at some point. By becoming more aware of the links between assertiveness and health, women can increase their understanding of and influence on both their own and others' behaviour.

Often, the links between assertiveness and health are implicit in women's lives. When asked, women on the Project said that assertiveness could help them to:

- Find a balance in life
- Feel more powerful
- Have a healthy mind, body and spirit
- Celebrate their culture and their strengths
- Believe there are choices
- Express and take responsibility for their feelings
- Deal effectively with health professionals
- 'Listen' to what their bodies are telling them
- Choose and negotiate relationships
- Make the most of what they are
- Say 'I need help'
- Value their bodies and eat the right food for them
- Find more time, more space and less stress
- Relax
- Take an interest in life
- Ask for information from health professionals
- Feel confident in taking important decisions
- Ask for a choice of treatments
- Choose a lifestyle that is right for them

- Feel good about themselves and value a self worth asserting

- Deal with conflicts in family or work

- Face up to contradictions in their lives and relationships

These answers show that women's definitions of health are broader than the standard medical model, which contrasts health with disease or sickness. Health encompasses emotional needs; attitudes and behaviours; political, social, and geographical environments; institutional policies and practices; and issues of race, sex, culture, class, sexuality, age and disability.

Assertiveness helps women firstly to recognise that they have a self worth asserting – that their needs and desires are valid and valuable. It can then help women to gain the skills needed to make their voices heard. These skills might include making firm requests, setting limits, giving and receiving compliments and criticisms, expressing and managing emotions, thinking positively, and using appropriate body language.

Assertiveness can help women feel that they have choices, and the right to explore their health even while constrained by any limitations that are placed on them. As such, it is part of wider women's health work, which supports women who are actively trying to make changes in themselves, their relationships, the environment, and policies and practices affecting their lives.

Why assertiveness and sexual health?

Some of the exercises in this book focus on sexual health in order to help women to think about and explore their sexuality. The World Health Organization (WHO) defines sexual health as:

> the integration of the physical, emotional, intellectual and social aspects of sexual being in ways that are enriching and that enhance personality, communication and love.
>
> (*AIDS action*, March 1991, 13:1)

Exercises on sexual health are scattered throughout the handbook. This is to encourage groups to look at sexual health as part of any work on assertiveness training and health, rather than something separate.

Who this handbook is for

Speaking out is for women who work with, or are involved in, groups of women in local communities – youth workers, community workers, community education tutors, HIV/AIDS workers, health promotion workers, paid or unpaid outreach workers. It has been written mainly for women who have already had some, but not necessarily extensive, experience of running groups.

Finding your way around this book

Speaking out is divided into five main sections.

Planning and facilitating

This provides a basic overview of how to work with groups, and some of the issues that you will need to consider: the kinds of experience and support needed; which women to ask and how to get them to come; practical arrangements; setting aims and objectives; thinking about ground rules; equal opportunities issues; potential problems; evaluation.

Frameworks

This offers suggestions for putting exercises together to develop sessions or courses, and gives three examples of combinations which have worked well in the past.

Exercise section I for all women's group

This section provides general exercises on assertiveness and health, grouped in themed sub-sections. Many of them suggest activities which are then followed by a group discussion, and highlight issues which groups may raise as a response. These exercises broadly tackle the need for assertiveness from a gender perspective, and do not explicitly deal with issues of race and culture.

Exercise section II for black women's groups

This section has been produced by and for black and minority ethnic women. Exercises in it are more discussion-based – a way of working which can be both familiar and risky. There are fewer ideas about the reactions exercises are likely to provoke: we hope that women will be able to adapt them to specific situations.

Throughout Section II, we have used the term 'black' to describe women from black and minority ethnic communities. (This was the term preferred by women developing these resources, and is used in a positive way to affirm the experiences of a group of people who have in common discrimination or disadvantage because of their skin colour or cultural differences.) You or the groups you work with may feel that you want to change some of the wording or assumptions of the exercises.

Although the section has been developed by and for black and minority ethnic women using a self-organising, community approach and with the assumption that women will have had similar experiences, this does not mean that if you're working with white or mixed groups it will not be relevant, stimulating and informative.

In both exercise sections, some exercises have photocopiable handouts which appear at the end of each group of exercises. These can be adapted and changed to fit the needs of individual groups.

Resources

On page 214 is a list of the resources used on the Project. These are divided into three main areas:

- Planning and facilitating
- For all women's groups
- For black women's groups

The list isn't intended to be comprehensive, but will give you some idea of the sorts of resources available.

You may also want to use *Every woman's health* (HEA 1993). With information and activities on all aspects of women's health, and detailed resource lists on specific subject areas, it's a useful companion to *Speaking out*.

In addition, the HEA's Health Promotion Information Centre will be able to help you search for both information on specific subject areas and for particular groups.

Planning and facilitating

This section looks at the practicalities involved in setting up assertiveness and women's health groups. It includes guidance on: getting women's groups together; developing course structures and programmes; setting ground rules; and evaluation. It also covers what kind of support you may need for yourself, and 'troubleshooting' problems.

There are a number of handouts and suggestions for ways of doing things which we hope you will find useful. Dip into the handbook and take what you need.

What is facilitating about?

This resource has been designed for women who already have some experience of working on health issues with groups of women. Generally, to be effective, facilitators need good everyday communication skills. These skills will need to be evaluated by the women you work with, however.

Your own group work and health experiences can be important to the group process. How you use these experiences will depend on your facilitative style, and how women in your group see you. Some facilitators prefer to be seen as 'tutors', sharing skills and knowledge about their subject. Others create a more informal, shared learning experience, in which they are no different from the women they work with. This can be a great advantage in terms of building up trust, and supporting and developing the group and individual women. On the down side, it can be hard to set realistic professional boundaries on the demands made on facilitators by women in the group.

Whichever way you work, the first step is to assess your style by evaluating and learning from past group experiences.

You could look at the following issues.

1   What you do and with whom. Who attends? Does this

reflect the make-up of the community? Do women take part? Which women? How and why?

2 Whether you provide choices and accessible information. Do you offer what women want in the way that they want it? What are the limitations placed on you?

3 Whether you listen to and hear what women are saying. Do you provide appropriate feedback? What feedback do you ask for from the group? How? What do you get?

4 Whether the group itself is supportive towards all women. How do you encourage this? Are women comfortable and at ease? How do you know? How are difficulties resolved?

It is important to understand non-verbal feedback – women leaving, or not turning up, feelings you pick up, and so on.

Support for facilitators

Where can you get help with ideas, creative ways of working, ways of evaluating effectiveness, or making groups more accessible to different women in different settings?

You might like to think about the following suggestions.

1 Talk over what you want to do with someone you trust. You may want to work through issues of personal development and consider your own strengths, limitations and boundaries.

2 Get involved in relevant networks and contacts to build your confidence and identify your level of awareness about different health issues and needs of different groups of women.

3 Work with someone more experienced or confident in working in a particular way or with particular groups.

4 Become part of a 'self-help' support group with other women group workers and encourage this approach to women's development work. You will be able to exchange information and ideas about ways of working: for example, dealing with distress, insensitivity and offensive remarks and behaviour.

A self-help approach will help you see any difficulties you are having as a learning process and will give you support outside the group you are facilitating.

What kind of groups?

Getting a group together

You may already have a group in mind with which to use this handbook. Here are some guidelines that we have found useful for bringing groups together.

Open groups

'Open' events are where the facilitator and/or the sponsoring organisation (a college of further education, for example) choose a venue and a time, and advertise locally for women to come along. Some of the work undertaken in the Project began in this way. One of the best ways of 'recruiting' for these groups is by word of mouth, directly to potential participants and through workers who can pass the information on to interested women.

Follow this up by putting leaflets and posters in libraries, schools, shop windows (you'll need to ask for permission first!), women's centres, community centres, youth clubs, GPs' surgeries, accommodation (including hostels) and groups for older women and women with disabilities. Local press and radio can also be useful in announcing when events are to take place.

Existing groups

You can work on assertiveness and health with existing groups: parent and toddler groups, access courses/groups at the local college or community centres, youth groups, oral history groups, creative writing groups, churches, temples or mosques, cultural festivals, lesbian support groups, groups run by a local well woman's centre, classes for English as a second language, or any other women's social, learning or friendship groups. In existing groups, women will already know each other, which can be an advantage. Offering to facilitate a one-off session may give you a way in to these settings. Women will often come back to you asking for more.

Formal groups

A series of sessions or a course can also be offered to women through local education authority (LEA) adult education classes, the Workers Educational Association (WEA), or through a local health promotion unit. You would need to negotiate such provision with the local management of these agencies.

Which health issues?

This depends on how you see health and how you want to work on health, sexual health and assertiveness. See the next section, *Frameworks*, for ways of assessing and working with groups on particular issues, or with particular groups of women.

Practical arrangements

Below are some practical considerations relating to developing and organising assertiveness and health groups.

Publicity

You should organise publicity in advance, usually either in the form of leaflets (including booking forms) or posters. The title and visual images are often key factors in attracting women to groups of this kind, so think carefully about who you want to attract.

The following are some examples of titles used by women involved in the Project for their publicity (many women preferred not to use the term 'assertiveness', since some find it off-putting, or too intimidating): *Women's well-being and assertiveness; Sharing and gathering; Well? Well!; Time for ourselves/ Introduction to health; Helping ourselves to health; Confidence building/ Health in middle years/Hersay; Time for ourselves: thinking about health; Women's health day/Health and wellness; Women's health development; Relationships and choices and who am I?*

Once you have generated an interest through your publicity, you will need to organise the following details. Do try to think and plan ahead for the varying needs of the different women who may attend and, if possible, speak to them about their requirements during the planning stage.

Time and date

Ensure that both time and date are convenient for the women who will attend and that, where possible, they can be reviewed at the start of the course. Consider, for example, bus times, dark nights, arranging transport, school hours and work hours. When setting the date try to avoid important religious festivals which may prevent women from attending. (Your local library may be able to provide you with more information.)

Advance information from participants

Use the publicity to provide information on access – availability and location of ramps, accessible toilets and so on. Ask women to indicate any special needs on their booking form – transport, special diet, childcare, signer, helper, seating etc.

Venue

Select a women-only space, if possible. Try to make sure that the venue is accessible and attractive to all women who want to attend, and that the attitude of others using the venue will not be detrimental to the women attending (people making derogatory or undermining comments about women, for example).

Seating

Try to ensure seating is comfortable and easy to move if you want to break into small groups, or if you need to make space for wheelchairs. Provide cushions for women who might need them.

Toilets

Check that adequate toilet facilities are available for women with disabilities and that there are disposal units for incontinence pads, etc.

Room preparation

The room should be big enough to allow the group to split into smaller groups to talk and not be overheard. Make sure that any equipment you need is available, that you will not be disturbed during the sessions (particularly important if you are dealing with sensitive issues), and that lighting and acoustics are good. Brighten a dull room with posters and flowers and, if possible, have comfortable chairs and a carpet or rug on the floor.

Numbers

Assess how many women you can take in the groups and decide how you will ensure that women who don't get a place, but who are interested, may be catered for later. Around 12 is a good number to work with, but up to 20 may work in some situations. Women can easily split into smaller discussion groups.

Childcare

Creche facilities (on site, preferably) are almost always essential for women with children. You should indicate in any publicity material or booking form whether there will be a charge.

An alternative is to fund women to find their own childminder.

Food

Consider whether you will provide food or if women will be asked to provide their own. Many groups bring food to share. If you are providing it, make sure that you know what dietary and cultural requirements there are from information on the booking form.

Food is an important way of promoting health and well-being and for recognising, and valuing different cultures, so do consider employing women from the local community to do the catering and ensure that they are clear about particular dietary requirements.

Make sure drinks are available throughout the event and provide caffeine- and sugar-free drinks as well as tea and coffee.

Finally

Be clear and specific about what you are offering, who you are and what organisation, if any, you represent. What can women expect to get out of attending a group of this kind? Where can you be contacted if participants need to get in touch with you for further details? Will you charge a fee for course attendance?

Ensure that women know how to get a place on the course or in the group and that your publicity welcomes all women regardless of age, ethnic origin, disability or sexual preference, unless you are working specifically with particular groups.

Use the checklist on p. 16 to make sure than you've covered everything.

Participation issues

Women do or do not attend groups for a number of reasons. It is important to consider these reasons and find ways of addressing them.

It can be demoralising to find that after putting a lot of energy into organising a course or event no one turns up or that the women who do come do not actually get involved. This might be because what you are doing:

- is not relevant or appropriate from the participants' point of view;

- is not accessible, inspiring, fun or attractive enough;

- does not take into account transport difficulties/childcare needs/costs incurred;

- does not fit in with their current priorities, or cannot compete with the other demands placed on their time;

- does not allay anxieties about what the experience might be like.

Many women care for young children or adult dependants, work in or outside the home, are lone parents without additional support, and have conflicting demands placed on their time. Others might feel that joining an assertiveness and health group, or meeting to address health issues, is threatening.

It might be appropriate to consider different ways of 'reaching out' or encouraging women to take part. This may have particular relevance for extending work within black or minority ethnic communities, or other marginalised groups. It is important to be very clear about what you are trying to achieve through your group work, and to make it as accessible as possible.

Within an existing group, it may be useful to look at some of the difficulties that may prevent particular groups of women taking part in health groups or events; and how the group may want to work with this in mind.

Catering for different communication needs

Women working with minority ethnic groups may find themselves dealing with two or more languages and dialects. Work with women with hearing difficulties and learning difficulties may involve using sign language as a way of communicating. This presents a real challenge to facilitators, but can also provide motivation to develop and use effective communication skills.

If you are planning to do some work with such groups, you will need to decide with the women (or a co-worker who knows the group) which main language(s) or means of communication the group will use and who will be interpreting. Interpreters should ideally be involved in any planning sessions.

It will help everyone if you keep language clear and use simple ways of communicating – pictures, cartoons and images, or simple statements, sayings and poems, for example.

You could split women up to work in groups of similar language. After the activity, you could have a brief feedback to the main group, to find out how it went.

Encourage the group to see that explaining, interpreting and clarifying what is happening are invaluable ways of promoting everyone's well-being and are not wasting time! Time spent in this way fosters good communication.

You could also think about using audio-visual resources in group work – most of the handouts and worksheets could be recorded on tape, and played back with appropriate spacing. This might prove useful for women with visual difficulties or for those who aren't used to using written material.

Offer the participants choices about how they might like to work. Suggestions could include using pictures and drawings, and communicating through symbols, mime, movement, touching and hugging, and any ways they themselves suggest.

Aims and objectives

Whether you are running a one-session introduction to assertiveness and health, a ten-session course, a weekend or weekday residential course, or whatever combination suits you and the group, you need to have a clear idea of your aims and objectives. These should be based on what women, any sponsoring organisations, and you yourself want to work on. Once you have established this, you can work out a more detailed structure (see the next section, *Frameworks*).

There are various ways of assessing women's expectations of assertiveness groups or courses, starting with simple questions such as, 'What do you want from this session/day/group?' Some of these methods are set out on page 40 onwards. You might like to use one or more of these exercises at the beginning of a course or group.

Developing a clear purpose

You need to be very clear about your purpose or aim. Knowing what you want to achieve with the group will enable you to plan and prepare more easily. You can then ensure that the exercises you use will fit your overall intention. The session will run more smoothly if you and the group are aware of the intended outcome.

Defining your objectives can also help you to set boundaries, and perhaps negotiate between what you want, what women want, and the requirements of any sponsoring organisation.

A personal action plan will help you clarify your ideas. You could either use or adapt the plan shown on pages 17–18.

On pages 19–20 there are two examples of aims and objectives developed by Project facilitators. You may get an idea from these of the difference between an overall aim (a general statement of intent) and an objective (a more specific statement indicating intended outcomes) and how you might write your own for or with the group you will be working with. Fill in the aims and objectives form on page 21 and keep for future reference.

Ground rules

There are many different ways of approaching ground rules or setting boundaries for a group. They are a good opportunity to find ways of working together and learning about each other. By working through ground rules, we can learn about our personal needs and differences. (For specific exercises on setting ground rules see exercise group II.)

There are four main areas that need to be identified, discussed and agreed upon.

1 *Confidentiality of shared personal experiences.*

2 *Supporting each other.* (It is good to look as a group at how you could do this, for example by listening to and respecting everyone's contributions.)

3 *Dealing with conflict, offence, etc.* Facilitators should assertively challenge comments or behaviour which are insensitive, cause offence or are discriminatory. Such difficult behaviour might be resolved by facilitators 'setting the scene' before difficulties arise. Acknowledge that everyone makes assumptions, but stress that dealing with this can be a learning process. You need to make clear that it is the group's responsibility to decide what to do about conflict, infringements of the ground rules, and insensitivity.

4 *Practical concerns,* such as smoking, breaks for drinks and timekeeping.

Groups may feel more 'together' as a result of negotiating and establishing their own ground rules. On pages 22–4 are some examples of ground rules used in the Project, which you might find useful to give out as handouts to provoke discussion.

Equal opportunities for everyone

Equal opportunities is about providing chances for all participants to benefit fully from a group or course, enabling women to promote their own and others' health and well-being, both within groups and outside them. This requires a genuine understanding of the kinds of inequalities that exist in everyday life for particular groups of people.

Good equal opportunities practice places responsibility on facilitators and group members to find ways of providing access and equality for all women. This can be encouraged by working through ground rules. However, individual women have to move beyond the slogans and rhetoric and begin to take personal responsibility for developing good practice by examining and understanding the way in which their value judgements influence their attitudes and behaviour.

As a facilitator, you need to be aware of the ways in which your own attitudes to others' situations, and even your way of working, can limit the opportunities available to other women to take responsibility for their health or express their health needs for themselves. Facilitators need to develop ways of working that acknowledge, explore and deal with assumptions, judgements and stereotypes. Usually, the best way to do this is by developing ground rules at the outset (see exercise group 11). This will help group members to avoid uncomfortable, uneasy or even distressing situations. You could also look out for opportunities to develop your own awareness (through training, outside support, and so on).

Facilitators can contribute to an equal-opportunity process in groups by spending some time on developing a framework for group activities. This can be an extension of the ground rules process. You might want to consider some of the following areas.

1 Drawing out some positive attitudes or ways in which women want to work towards valuing and understanding different experiences and perspectives in the group.

2 Looking at experiences women have had in any women's groups in the past. What did and what did not promote equal opportunities?

3 Exploring feelings and attitudes about potential conflict arising in the group.

Equal opportunities and working on sexual health

Certain sexual health topics may be sensitive and uncomfortable for groups and facilitators, but work on sexual health can also show how equal opportunities is practised. Group members can be helped to accept different sexualities and not to judge people according to their sexual orientation or experiences. Facilitators should be aware of their own attitudes and anxieties about dealing with sexual health, and need to be open-minded and fairly well-informed. The following issues need to be considered.

Information

You need to have a basic knowledge of sexual health (how HIV is spread and not spread, for example) so that you are able to deal with any questions and/or prejudices. (See *Resources* section.)

Facilitators don't need to be experts, nor should groups assume that you are. You will have to make sure that you are comfortable with saying 'I don't know but I can find out', or referring women to other sources of information. Sometimes other group members may be able to provide information or someone may find out and bring it to the next session.

Spend some time thinking through the issues that may come up about HIV/AIDS and other sexually transmitted diseases or sexual health problems. You can get advice from colleagues; some local health promotion units may have specialist HIV workers who can help. You could also contact local family planning clinics, health advisers at genito-urinary medicine (GUM) clinics, GPs' surgeries, counselling services, gay and lesbian helplines or groups, and so on.

Most of us are uncomfortable about discussing some aspects of sex and sexuality. You could think about working with a co-facilitator to share knowledge and experience and discuss issues that come up. You could also talk to colleagues – to work through the issues, learn about new resources, and gain confidence.

Facilitators have found that women in their groups are their own experts, and will have enough knowledge and experience to keep groups going for months! Your skill as a facilitator is important in drawing out and encouraging women to find new ways of thinking and behaving which will be of benefit to them. In this way, women can help each other explore ways of loving that encompass a range of sensual and sexual activities.

Groups

Not all women will have had experience of talking about their sexual health, and some may be constrained from doing so by cultural norms or values. It is essential that facilitators make clear right from the start that women are likely to be of differing sexualities and communities and will have different experiences and likes and dislikes. Stress that everyone's contribution will be valued and accepted, and be prepared to challenge sensitively any obvious heterosexism and other prejudices if they occur.

Trust takes time to build up in groups so do make sure that you allow plenty of opportunity for women to get to know each other. Be aware of any differences of opinion which may create difficulties within the group.

Encourage the group not to make assumptions about each other or women generally: that they are in a relationship; that they are heterosexual; that they are/are not sexually active. Remember that just because women do not overtly state that they are lesbian or bisexual in the early stages of the group does not mean that they are not. (Some married women may identify as lesbian or bisexual, for example.)

Areas of concern

Some sexual health resources tend to concentrate on women's sexual body parts and describe sexuality in the context of reproduction, instead of seeing it as a much broader area of our lives. Women's position in society greatly affects the way we feel about ourselves, our self-esteem and our self-confidence. In order to address assertiveness and health, we need firstly to be aware of the context in which we are living: for example, the influence of history, religion and male-dominated institutions such as the media. Our sexual health is certainly not just about our reproductive systems.

Be sensitive to the groups you are working with and any differences in cultural background, beliefs, age, sexuality, ability and class. Don't choose sexual health issues or use materials that may be relevant only to heterosexual women.

Try to be sensitive about the use of language in the group. 'Foreplay', for instance, implies that other sexual activity is just a preliminary to penetrative sex.

Potential problems

Example 1

What happens if you have to challenge someone's (or someone challenges your own) behaviour or lack of awareness?

You need to find ways of offering group members and

yourself a chance to address potential difficulties of this nature before they arise, and to acknowledge them and deal with them constructively. It is vital to create an environment where women are not discouraged from opening their mouths for fear of offending someone. Equally, avoid situations where every group member, including the facilitator, is looking to the one woman with disabilities, or the one black woman or lesbian in the group, to be the 'expert' or for approval in what they say or do.

Suggested problem-solving approach

- Introduce ground rules as an opportunity for the group to work through, learn from and support each other.

- Agree with the group positive ways of acknowledging differences in order to develop an understanding of them. Group members may feel that they don't want to work with women who are unable to agree with group resolutions and boundaries.

Example 2

At some point in your personal development as a facilitator you may be faced with having to acknowledge the real or potential blocks in working with groups of women different from yourself. This could be white women working with black women, black women working with white women, able-bodied women working with women with disabilities, or lesbians working with heterosexual women. How can we work through this process?

Suggested problem-solving approach

You could adapt the following questions, used on the Project, to raise the following questions with the group.

- What do participants want/not want from their time together?

- What are the blocks/difficulties? What are the positive ways forward?

Evaluation

Evaluation needs to be taken into account from the very beginning of the planning process, when you find out about participants' expectations. If these expectations have changed over time, this is an interesting point in its own right. Evaluation need not be complicated. It is merely a way of checking whether you are meeting your original aims.

Be clear about why you are doing evaluation.

- Is it to check out how participants are feeling or thinking about the group?

- Do you require feedback on structure and presentation to guide you in planning future courses or groups?

- Does your organisation require feedback? If so, what specifically? How will it be used?

- Does the group itself require a way of consolidating and reviewing what it has done in order to see whether it has achieved its objectives?

These different reasons will require different methods of evaluation.

- Through discussion with individual group members or the group as a whole.

- Listing on a flipchart or board how participants feel about their progress (a simple way of doing this is to ask women to identify one positive and one negative thing so far).

- Exercises or questionnaires for participants to complete. (A number of these examples are given on pages 25–32. Some (examples 1 and 2) can be used for either individual sessions or the course as a whole.)

It is better to develop your own evaluation methods, appropriate to your group. What do you want to know? What kind of questions will enable you to find this out? You might want to ask participants some of the following questions.

- Do you have any comments on the course structure?

- Which areas have been most useful to you?

- Which have been least useful?

Finally, don't make a meal of evaluation! The simplest ways often yield the most information. Most people want to learn, not keep going over what they have learned, useful as this can be, so do ensure that the evaluation procedures you use enable learning to be consolidated and extended.

Below are some examples of the kind of feedback you might get on courses.

Participant feedback

Body image session needed lots more time! The drawings encouraged women to be very open about how they saw themselves and some very interesting discussions evolved regarding shape. (This session was drawn to a close with a positive handout entitled 'I am me'.)

I have learned to listen to other people.
I am more confident with people in authority.
I am able to express myself more confidently and more clearly. I have learnt to listen more, both to myself (my body language), and to what other people are saying about me.

Basket of sexual health – this went well and I found it interesting and informative. There was a reluctance by some who found it difficult to handle the items, e.g. condom, coil and contraceptive sponge.

Brought together different cultures.
Stimulating conversation.
Not inhibiting – respect for each other's cultures.

Facilitator feedback

Verbal feedback has been fairly positive.
Rooms chosen not comfortable.
Times were difficult.
Role play unpopular.
Everyone surprised at how relaxed they felt!
All would like support.

After the course one woman successfully attended a test for communication skills at the training centre. Before the course she was often sick or didn't turn up for such tests.

All women attended the group each session.
Great deal of support between the women.
A lot of sharing of very personal feelings and experiences.
Women gave feedback spontaneously as well as when asked.

Checklist for planning a group

1   Is the group open to all women?

How can I target particular groups of women who do not usually attend or might not have heard about this event – through networks or specific minority publications?

Have I checked that the date does not coincide with important religious or cultural festivals in various communities?

2   Have I thought about the practical and emotional needs of women with disabilities/special needs, and asked women what specific help they might need – transport, helper, signer, seating, or diet?

Have I considered how I might need to adapt the programme to accommodate their needs?

3   Have I sorted out childcare arrangements?

4   Have I asked women about their dietary requirements and organised the catering (if needed)?

Personal action plan

- What do I want to achieve?

- Why do I want to do this?

- What are my specific goals or objectives?

- How will I achieve them?

- Who else will I need to involve?

▶

- What other resources do I need?

- What might stop me?

- What do I need to do first?

- What is my timescale?

- How will I know I have been successful?

Aims and objectives: example 1

Aim

To introduce assertiveness and how it is linked to health.

Objectives

- To build self-confidence and self-esteem.
- To clarify, demystify and define assertiveness.
- To be aware of non-assertive behaviour and how this affects health.
- To make links between assertiveness and a holistic view of health.
- To introduce some assertiveness skills:
  - saying no
  - criticism
  - asking for what I want
  - anger and stress.

Aims and objectives: example 2

Aim

To provide a community-based women's health course for women who wish to increase their knowledge, confidence and skills.

Objectives

- To give women the opportunity to meet and talk with other women about women's health needs and other related issues.

- To develop women's knowledge, skills and confidence during group discussions.

- To enable women to explore how their attitudes towards their bodies, health and health care may be influenced by social, cultural and economic factors.

- To encourage women to explore how their worries and prejudices may be shaped by their own experiences.

- To develop an awareness of how women may help and support each other by sharing their skills and experiences.

My aims and objectives

Fill in the following form and use it to develop your aims and objectives.

Whole course

1 What do you as a facilitator want to achieve?

2 What do you think participants want from a group like this? (Check this out with participants.)

3 What does your sponsoring organisation expect?

Individual sessions

1 What do you want to achieve?

2 What do participants want to achieve?

3 What will they get?

Remember to write the above as statements of outcomes you and the participants want as a result of involvement in the course or group.

Ground rules: example 1

- No smoking (There was only one smoker and she agreed not to smoke for this workshop.)
- Confidentiality
- Responsibility to the group
- Timekeeping (As facilitators we had to look at timekeeping. It was clear that the women were not going to be able to keep to the planned timetable and also that they wanted to finish early on the Sunday. This was negotiated and agreed.)
- Tutors not to use jargon
- Accepting constructive criticism
- Willingness to share
- No offence when facilitator requests a participant to wind up

Review and build on ground rules weekly.

Ground rules: example 2

- Confidentiality
- Support – right to keep quiet
- Respect each other's opinions
- Don't tell others what to do
- Honesty
- Listen to others
- Show compassion when someone is upset
- Don't belittle others
- Welcome new people
- Avoid superiority
- Common language

Ground rules: example 3

- Warm, friendly, caring
- Confidentiality: keep personal information within the group
- You don't have to do things if you don't want to
- Don't judge
- You are responsible for your own learning
- Support each other
- Listen to others and don't talk over them
- Need for a closed room

Evaluation example 1

For use at the beginning of a course and throughout as a fun way of monitoring how people feel about themselves at different stages.

Participants are given a copy of *The confidence tree* handout (p. 26) and asked to put their name at the top. The facilitator can help by working through the cartoon and calling attention to particular favourite or contradictory characters.

Participants are asked to study the handout individually for a few minutes and to decide which character they feel most represents themselves in terms of self-confidence at the present time. They are asked to place a number one by that character.

Explain that the handout will be kept and used to chart personal development in confidence over the remaining weeks of the course.

Extra points of discussion raised by the handout:

- How our confidence ebbs and flows with particular situations and on particular days.

- How, when we are confident in something, we take it for granted.

- How we take more notice of the situations in which we are not confident than those in which we are confident.

The confidence tree

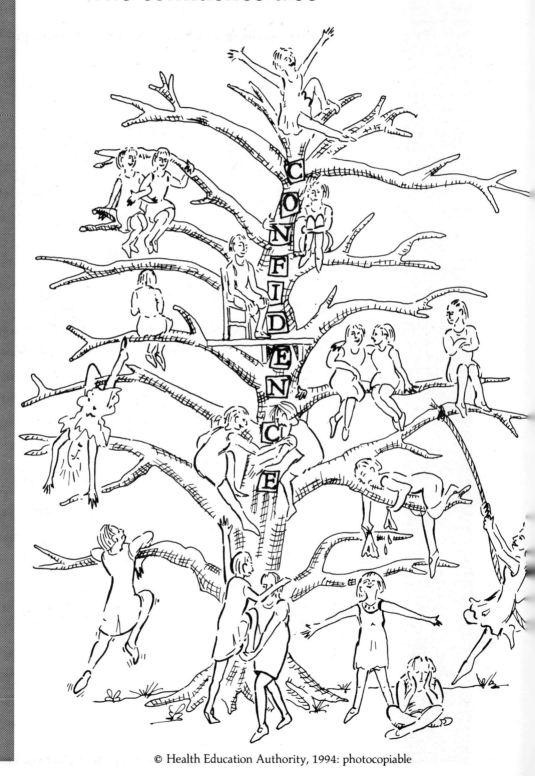

Evaluation example 2

Circle the words which show how you are feeling right now.

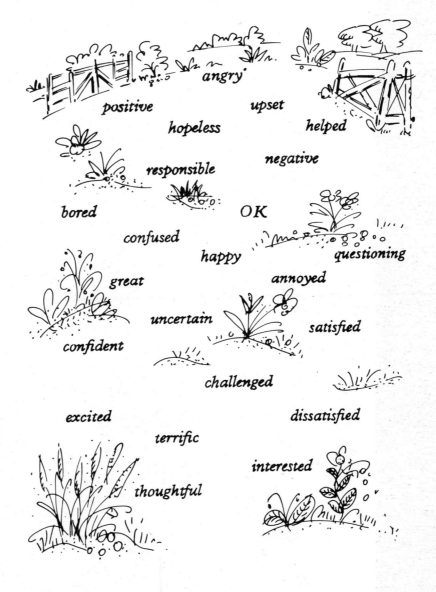

positive

angry

upset

hopeless

helped

responsible

negative

bored

OK

confused

happy

questioning

great

annoyed

uncertain

satisfied

confident

challenged

excited

dissatisfied

terrific

interested

thoughtful

Adapted from *Greater expectations* (LDA)

Evaluation example 3

The thing I liked best about today was . . .

The thing I did not like about today was . . .

Next time I hope to . . .

It would be a good idea if you included . . .

The most useful part of the day was . . .

Before the next session I will think about . . .

Evaluation example 4

Please indicate the value of each session by circling the numbers below.

Session (1)   NOT USEFUL 1 2 3 4 5 6 7 8 9 10 VERY USEFUL

Session (2)   NOT USEFUL 1 2 3 4 5 6 7 8 9 10 VERY USEFUL

Session (3)   NOT USEFUL 1 2 3 4 5 6 7 8 9 10 VERY USEFUL

Session (4)   NOT USEFUL 1 2 3 4 5 6 7 8 9 10 VERY USEFUL

Session (5)   NOT USEFUL 1 2 3 4 5 6 7 8 9 10 VERY USEFUL

Session (6)   NOT USEFUL 1 2 3 4 5 6 7 8 9 10 VERY USEFUL

Session (7)   NOT USEFUL 1 2 3 4 5 6 7 8 9 10 VERY USEFUL

Session (8)   NOT USEFUL 1 2 3 4 5 6 7 8 9 10 VERY USEFUL

Session (9)   NOT USEFUL 1 2 3 4 5 6 7 8 9 10 VERY USEFUL

Least useful session: please explain why briefly.

Most useful session: please explain why briefly.

Do you feel more able to use assertiveness skills as a result of this course?

Are you able to see links between assertiveness and health more clearly now? (Please expand your answer if possible.)

Did you relate the exercises to health situations . . .
- Most of the time?
- Some of the time?
- Not at all?

(Please circle one.)

Do you feel confident about working with groups of people in this way?

What, if anything, could have been left out?

What, if anything, could have been given more emphasis or included?

How will you be able to link assertiveness skills with health situations you face?

Any other comments:

Evaluation example 5

Please help us by filling in this form. Please be honest with your views and criticisms as this will help us when planning other courses.

The evaluation sheets are confidential, but feel free to write your name on the top if you wish to do so.

1   Overall, have you found the course useful? (Please tick one answer.)

Yes   No   Unsure

2   Has the course helped you in any of the following ways? (Please tick any you agree with.)

Given you practical skills

Explained why women lack confidence

Given you more confidence

Taught you techniques with which to practise becoming more confident

3   How have you found the course? (Please tick any you agree with.)

Useful

Supportive

Practical

Unhelpful

Confusing

Over your head

4   Do you think that you will be more confident in outside situations because of the course? (Please tick one answer.)

Yes   No   Unsure

▶

5   Was the course the right length? (Please tick one answer.)

Long enough

Too short

Too long

6   Have you enjoyed the course? (Please tick one answer.)

Yes   No   Unsure

7   Have you found other members of the group supportive? (Please tick one answer.)

Yes   No   No comment

8   How would you rate the course? (Please tick one answer.)

Very good

Good

Okay

Poor

Very poor

9   Please state anything else that you think should have been included in the course.

10 Please feel free to add any other comments about the course.

Frameworks

This section looks at how facilitators can use the exercises in *Speaking out* to develop sessions or courses. It won't plan them for you, but will give you some ideas about the issues you'll need to consider. It begins by outlining some general concepts and moves on to particular models for putting courses or sessions together. These are only suggestions: the groups you work with may well want to explore different combinations, or add exercises from elsewhere.

Meeting the needs of the group

Facilitators on the Project did this in different ways.

Beforehand

By developing a course or session outline and negotiating it with other colleagues before presenting it to the group for discussion and agreement at the first session. Often this is the only practicable way of going about things if the group cannot come together beforehand.

With the group

By having pre-course meetings, or setting aside time at the first meeting, where women brainstorm what they might want or need. Often, this means that there is a high degree of involvement right from the beginning of the planning process. You'll probably have to be quite flexible when using this approach: new needs may emerge, or women may not feel able to express needs before they know and trust the group. Not having everything planned out in advance can also be quite scary for the facilitator.

The first exercise group in Exercise section I *Styles and ways of working* provides a number of exercises to help facilitators gauge where groups are, and where they would like to go, with assertiveness, health and sexual health. The first exercise group in Exercise section II, *Taking part* (exercise group 10) covers facing what women want from groups and how to achieve it; and a later section, *Assertiveness and our own health* (13) suggests a number of exercises which map out what women understand by assertiveness and its relevance to them. You might want to combine some of these with other exercises in an introductory session.

Facilitators need to ensure that the programme is flexible and allows women's needs to be met. You may, however, have to balance this with leading the group in identifying and drawing out the links between health and assertiveness if women have never worked on these areas before.

Choosing exercises

Read through *Planning and facilitating* (especially the action plans in *Aims and objectives*) and any materials from the *Resources* section which you think might be useful. You will then need to outline:

- what your own needs from the group are;

- what your organisation's (if any) needs are;

- what the needs are of the women you will be working with (which you may either know from talking to women at the first session, or assess independently).

These might be quite easy to identify: perhaps you are running a 12-week adult education class for older women who don't have much experience of assertiveness training; or working with a mixed group of young women with learning difficulties who need to gain assertiveness skills. Whatever your situation, it's important to be as clear as possible at this stage.

You'll then need to look through Exercise sections I and II to identify which exercises might suit the group. Each sub-section has an introduction outlining the scope of the exercises in it, and each exercise has a 'Suitable for' entry giving details of the kinds and stages of groups with which it has proved successful. (Exercises in section I also have an 'Issues raised' entry outlining some of the potential benefits and risks of using them.)

You'll need to bear in mind that section II exercises are more discussion-based. You might want to moderate these with more activity-based exercises from section I.

Carefully read through the exercises you think might be appropriate. The following questions may help you clarify whether you could use them.

- How appropriate is the title of the exercise? Do you want to change it?

- Is the purpose realistic? Could it be adapted or improved?

- Is the method clear? Could it be adapted or improved?

- Approximately how long will the exercise take?

- When could you use it? Are there any issues that will have to be covered before you can use it? Are there any issues that it will raise that can be worked through in another exercise?

- What does the group need for this exercise to be successful?

You'll need to keep timings in mind. As a rough guide, use no more than two or three exercises in any half-day block; or one or two for a two-hour session.

Working out an order

Both Exercise sections are loosely structured in an order which facilitators have found useful in the past: moving from introductory, foundation-laying work on the nature and purpose of the group; through specific work on how women see themselves and others; to tackling more sensitive issues and the application of assertiveness work to women's lives. You might want to follow these thematic structures, but there are also a number of practical points which facilitators have found useful in the past:

- It's important to begin and end with some kind of game or exercise to get everyone talking to each other and feeling comfortable. (Obviously, this will be easier in an established group.) Although *Speaking out* includes some exercises which could be used as ice-breakers or ending exercises, there are many more in *Women together* (see *Resources* section).

- Ground rules need to be established as soon as possible. (See page 9, pages 22–4, and pages 158–62.)

- Make sure that sensitive areas (such as sexual health) are not put either right at the beginning of a group's life (when women may not feel 'safe' enough with each other to discuss very personal issues) or at the end (when there may not be time to ensure that whatever comes up is dealt with adequately).

Suggested models for courses or groups

These draw on both Exercise sections, and most offer at least two choices for suitable exercises in each case. You will have to assess the appropriateness of each exercise for your group.

The links between assertiveness and health

Aim

To enable women to identify how assertiveness can be used to enhance their health and well-being. This kind of session is the ideal introduction to the relevance of assertiveness. You could offer it to parent and toddler groups, friendship groups or youth groups.

First exercise

Becoming more healthy and assertive (5D)

What is assertiveness? (1F)

Making connections (13B)

Good for enabling women to establish for themselves the link between assertiveness and health, and to set the scene for the session.

Second exercise

Rights and choices (7B)

The implications of assertiveness (13D)

A practical opportunity for women to discuss the impact of assertiveness on their lives and the choices it can enable them to make.

Self-esteem and health

Aim

To provide a one-day programme for older women exploring how self-esteem can affect their sense of well-being and ability to make choices.

Many older women face some kind of health issue influenced by their age. This can range from feeling more tired, and experiencing specific health problems such as osteoporosis or arthritis, to dealing with loss and grief. Coupled with this are attitudes to growing older. Many older women are also facing life as carers, or are learning to be cared for or living alone for the first time. Courses like this one offer older women opportunities to explore how to develop and maintain a new and different sense of self, and also provide much-needed support and reassurance.

First exercise

Haystack (2C)

Warm-up around differences (12A)

Great for getting women to begin to look at what they value about themselves and for getting groups working well together.

Second exercise

Self-esteem and health (2A)

How we talk to ourselves (3A)

Enables women to begin to explore the links between higher self-esteem and better health and well-being. *Self-esteem and health* will promote discussion; *How we talk to ourselves* offers practical ways forward.

Third exercise

TV characters (2B)

Images of women (4A)

Y'a ba'an b' y'a n'a! (17C)

Offers opportunities to look at why self-esteem can vary at different points in women's lives.

Fourth exercise

Feeling good about ourselves (3B)

Working on ourselves (17D)

A chance for women to look practically at what they might do to increase their self-esteem.

Assertiveness and health

Aim

To provide a six-session course for young women, giving them an opportunity to identify the relevance of assertiveness to them. This type of format is ideal for use with groups that meet regularly anyway – in youth clubs, for example. Each session will probably last between one and two hours.

Session 1

Becoming more healthy and assertive (5D)

Making connections (13B)

Self-esteem and health (2A)

Session 2

Images of women (4A)

How do others see me? How do I see myself? (12E)

The roles and stereotypes ascribed to women by the media and other people.

Session 3

TV characters (2B)

Good for looking at self-esteem from a distance – identifying what it is in other people.

Session 4

Relationships (6N)

Ending relationships (6S)

Thinking about sexual relationships and the areas which are often the most difficult to face.

Session 5

Saying no (7C)

Follows on from the previous session, which may have provided useful 'real life' situations to practise saying no in.

Session 6

Rights and choices (7B)

Raising the issues (14A)

Good practical exercises to round off.

Exercise section I
For all women's groups

1 Styles and ways of working: introducing assertiveness and health

The following exercises may be useful at the beginning of a course or session. They will help you find out what women expect and need from the group, and what they understand about both health and assertiveness.

The first five exercises are fun ways of brainstorming the kinds of issues that women want to look at. They present you with a variety of ways to encourage women to identify subject areas – either individually, in small groups, or in the large group.

The remaining exercises cover defining assertiveness and its relevance to group members – and some of the reasons why women may find it difficult to behave assertively.

1A Quilt

EXERCISE

Materials
A number of cut-out hexagon shapes, pens.

Method
1   Give each woman a number of hexagon shapes. Ask them to write down what they consider to be the issues involved in assertiveness and health, one on each shape.

2   Gather up the shapes and put them all together, clustering them as appropriate, for example, around sexual health, self-esteem, etc. You can then follow the sessions accordingly.

You can also do this exercise on stickers and then stick them on to a piece of flipchart paper.

1B Cards

E X E R C I S E

Materials
Write down some issues which may prove difficult for women (perhaps taboo subjects) on separate cards.

Method
Write the cards in advance. Ask group members to choose what they do/do not want to deal with. Women could indicate their choices by raising their hands, or anonymously (using ticks or crosses on the cards) to enable women who might be worried about self-disclosure in the early stages of a group – concerning, for example, sexual difficulties, lesbian relationships, sexual abuse or violence in relationships – to explore their feelings.

1C Snowball

E X E R C I S E

Materials
Sheets of flipchart paper, each one with an appropriate title heading, such as stress/anxiety, women's health, confidence, menopause, etc.

Method
1 Split women up into small groups, preferably by a random method such as numbers or colours (go round the circle and number each woman (1, 2, 3, 4; 1, 2, 3, 4) then put all the 'ones' in one group, the 'twos' in another etc.).

2 Give each group a flipchart sheet with a title heading and ask them to discuss that heading. Their task is to identify what they would want as a group from a session with that title, and to write/draw their ideas on flipchart paper. You should stress that you want ideas, not definitive answers, and that they can put down anything.

3 After a given length of time, swap the sheets between the groups, so each group gets a flipchart with a title heading that has already been worked on by a previous group. Each group adds anything important to them that is not already there.

4 At the end of the exercise, all the sheets should have been seen by every group. The result is a comprehensive collection of thoughts, ideas and needs that women have identified for themselves on a particular topic, which can act as a base from which to develop the course content.

1D Needs and expectations

EXERCISE

Purpose

To encourage participants to say what they expect to gain from the group, so their thoughts are focused and their agenda can be taken into account.

Materials

Flipchart paper, pens.

Method

Ask women to call out issues that they want to look at, and what they might get out of the group. One woman should write down what others come up with.

The list generated when this exercise was used during the Project is shown below (items marked with an asterisk are specifically linked to health).

- Find what we enjoy
- Women's needs being taken into account by partner, relatives, e.g. daughters
- Being able to switch off mentally from other people's problems or responsibilities
- *Negotiating – communicating with others in a way that involves respect and co-operation – builds our health
- *Share our thoughts on health
- *Food and health
- How we can get time for ourselves – without feeling guilty
- *If you have half an hour to yourself, how can you use it for your health?
- *Weight – coping with it
- *Women as carers
- *Learning to give ourselves time
- Planning ahead
- Finance
- *Images of us being tidy and beautiful
- *How to tackle health professionals
- Feeling confident in our choices about our lives and/or finding the strength to make new choices

The facilitator could then 'group' issues together in particular 'areas'.

Issues raised

On the Project, women provided a lengthy list of what they were hoping to get out of the course. They said that being able to communicate more effectively would enhance their health. They also felt it was important that they gave time to themselves; each spoke of how she had to manage her time in order to get to the workshop, for example, organising childcare, rearranging other events, etc. This exercise generated such a lot of interest that it was extended beyond the time originally allocated to it.

1E Questions to consider

EXERCISE

Purpose

To enable participants to identify what they want from an assertiveness and health group.

Materials

A copy of handout 1A for each participant.

Method

1   Give each participant a copy of handout 1A and ask them to split up into pairs and discuss their thoughts on each question listed.

2   In the whole group, suggest that participants may gain the following from the group or course

   ● Understanding what assertiveness means

   ● Increased self-confidence and self-esteem

   ● Understanding why you might be unassertive

   ● Learning how to communicate feelings honestly and appropriately

   ● Assertiveness skills:

     – Saying no

     – Asking for what you want

     – Dealing with emotions

   ● Increased self-awareness

   ● Understanding what health means to you

   ● Becoming more healthy by becoming more assertive

   ● Becoming more capable of taking responsibility for your health and your life

Issues raised

The last two questions allow space for women to express any worries that could potentially get in the way of their learning. They also acknowledge that women often lead very hectic and demanding lives, and can feel guilty about taking time for themselves. Good discussion points, relevant to assertiveness and health, can therefore be developed from these apparently simple questions.

1F What is assertiveness?

EXERCISE

Purpose

- To clarify the differences between assertive and non-assertive behaviour.

- To set the scene for further exploration and practice in relating assertiveness to health.

Suitable for

Useful at the beginning of a course or group, and with women of all ages.

Materials

A copy of handout 1B for each participant.

For Variation 1, three sheets of flipchart paper.

For Variation 2, cards bearing statements beginning 'Being assertive is . . .', 'Being aggressive is . . .' and 'Being passive is . . .'. Use the examples in the handout to prepare the cards.

For Variations 3 and 4, large pieces of paper and pens (of at least two colours).

Method

Begin with an explanation of the need to identify what assertiveness means. A lot of behaviour that is called assertive may actually be aggressive, so you need to look at the difference between assertive, aggressive and passive behaviour.

Variation 1

1 Write up on a flipchart 'Assertiveness means'. Get the group to brainstorm examples, followed by a discussion about which are assertive and which might not be.

2 Do the same with 'Passiveness means', and 'Aggressiveness means'. Ask women to identify what behaviour might be 'indirect aggression'. Do any of the things they come up with fit into this category?

3   End the exercise by getting women to look at the definitions in the handout if they have not already done so. Compare these with what women have come up with themselves. Explain how this type of exercise helps to 'set the scene' for the group in looking at assertiveness and their health.

Variation 2

1   Lay all the cards (see Materials) out on a table or the floor and ask women to get into groups of twos or threes. Ask each group to pick one or more example from each category, and get them to discuss what the differences are between the categories of behaviour. Do they disagree with any of the statements?

2   Bring everyone back to the main group and ask each group to read out their cards and discuss their reactions to them.

Variation 3

1   Divide the group into three. Ask one group to write down what they think assertiveness means, the second group what aggressiveness means and the third what passiveness means. Everyone in the group should write something if they want to, but there should be as little discussion as possible.

2   Swap the sheets around so that each group now has another's piece of paper. Ask each group to discuss what the other group has come up with. Do they agree with it? Ask the groups to write any disagreement in a second colour next to the relevant statement.

3   In the main group identify what, if anything, groups didn't agree with. End the session with small groups giving two examples of statements that everyone agrees on.

Variation 4

1   Divide the group into threes and fours and give each group a large piece of paper divided into three columns with the headings 'Aggressive', 'Passive' and 'Assertive'. Ask women to list anyone in the media, on TV, soap operas, etc. who fits into these categories.

2   Bring women back to the main group and ask for feedback on who they put into which category and why.

This variation is harder than people think. People usually disagree about which character or person should go into which category. Some groups have the same person in different categories, showing that everyone behaves in all of these ways at various times. Most groups have found this exercise fun. It really brings home the characteristics of assertiveness. (Many thanks to Mid-Glamorgan Health Promotion Unit for giving us this variation.)

Issues raised

- This kind of exercise is a good introduction to assertiveness. It enables women to think about various different types of behaviour and what they mean, and shows them that they do have the knowledge they need in order to move on.

- In most groups it is difficult behaviour that is easier to describe, and assertive behaviour that provokes the most discussion.

1G Obstacles to assertiveness

E X E R C I S E

Purpose

To promote discussion on what prevents women being assertive.

Suitable for

Groups already familiar with issues around assertiveness and health.

Materials

Flipchart paper and pens.

Method

1 Write in the middle of a piece of flipchart paper, 'What prevents us being assertive even when we are clear about what we want?'

2 Ask women to give examples. Write them up as you go along.

Variation

Write the same question on the middle of a piece of flipchart paper and write the following statements around it.

- Wanting to be liked and approved of

- Not wanting to be a nuisance

- Others' insecurity

- Having to justify ourselves

- Stereotyped roles

- Pressure from family and friends

- Overreacting

- Fear of reprisal

- Media/advertising 'norms'

- Guilt

- Dislike of challenging other people

- Being seen as 'fussy'

- Being unsure whether what we want (to see a woman doctor or consultant, for example) is available

Discussion

You could centre a discussion around any of the things women come up with, or use any of the statements above. For example:

- **Guilt**
  Where, when and how is guilt implanted in us? Is it cultural? religious? Is it linked to gender? Why are some people harder on themselves than others? Does feeling guilty prevent us from living life to the full?

- **Stereotyped roles**
  Who are we as women – wives, lovers, mothers, sisters, etc? How do we feel about the roles allotted to us and what happens when we try to be assertive?

- **Others' insecurity**
  Do we take responsibility for others' insecurity and if so, why?

1A Questions to consider

1 What have you come for?

2 What do you hope to gain?

3 What have you left behind?

4 How do you feel about it?

1B What is assertiveness?

Definitions

Assertive behaviour enables people to act in their own best interests and stand up for their rights while also respecting the rights and feelings of others. It enables people to express both positive and negative feelings comfortably and without *undue* anxiety.

Aggressive behaviour is when people try to get what they want at all costs with no thought for the feelings of others – by bullying, being sarcastic, threatening or putting down other people. It can also involve less direct aggression by using manipulative and devious means such as emotional blackmail or flattery.

Passive behaviour is when people deny their rights and their personal feelings, which they rarely express openly. Needs are therefore seldom met, with a consequent loss of self-esteem. Typical behaviours are sighing, hinting, wishing and sulking.

Examples of assertive behaviour

- Being aware of your rights and acknowledging the rights of others
- Knowing what you really want – having a clear sense of direction
- Saying what you mean – and meaning what you say
- Rewarding yourself for achievement
- Loving yourself and others when you choose to love
- Knowing your own value
- Not being intimidated

- Having choices and breaking old ways of behaving
- Being able to negotiate
- Changing your mind
- Choice
- Being able to say no and not feel guilty
- Confidence
- Telling people confidently and clearly what you want, need, or prefer, without threatening or putting down others

Examples of aggressive behaviour

- Verbal abuse
- Putting people down
- Great, if I'm winning!
- Interrupting
- Uncontrolled responses
- Domination
- Being argumentative
- Not allowing other people to change
- Inappropriate anger
- Lack of consideration
- Bullying
- Domineering
- At the expense of someone else!
- Negation
- Threatening

Examples of indirectly aggressive or manipulative behaviour

- Deviousness
- Putting people down behind their backs
- Dishonesty
- Emotional blackmail

Examples of passive behaviour

- Fearing authority
- Knowing what you need but lacking the energy to claim it
- Being angry with yourself
- Doubting
- Feeling small
- Feeling outmanoeuvred
- Having no rights
- Always saying yes
- Trying to please others and not yourself
- Avoiding conflict
- Feeling humiliated
- Not putting yourself first
- Sitting on the fence

2 Self-esteem and confidence

Our self-esteem continually needs nourishing and nurturing if we are to become secure, healthy and assertive human beings. Low self-esteem or lack of self-worth can often lead to passive or aggressive behaviour. It is much more difficult to assert ourselves when we are feeling low and lack confidence and conviction. If we feel we don't have the right to say no we can't say it strongly; and we often put up with things we don't like because we feel other people's feelings are more important.

The following exercises give women an opportunity to work on self-esteem and confidence in assertiveness training and to look at where women get their sense of self-esteem/worth from. The exercises will help women identify and develop the positive qualities they already have but often do not acknowledge. This then gives women a firmer foundation from which to assert themselves.

2A Self-esteem and health

E X E R C I S E

Purpose

To acknowledge that high self-esteem is a starting point for assertiveness and health and that confidence is a by-product of this.

Suitable for

Introducing the above topics to a group. It is a particularly good exercise to use with young women, who may be just beginning to develop a sense of their adult 'self', and with older women, to explore what has influenced their sense of self and how it has changed.

Materials

Flipchart paper and pens. A copy of handout 2A for each woman.

Method

1   Ask women to pair up and think carefully about where they get their sense of self from – country of origin, culture, TV, media, history/'herstory', friends, partners, teachers, family, work and so on.

2   Bring women back into the main group and ask for feedback on what they came up with. Write this up on the flipchart.

3 Next, ask women in pairs to brainstorm words that come to mind when they think about self-esteem.

4 Write these up. As a group, try to come up with a definition of self-esteem that fits everyone's perceptions of it.

Discussion

1 Develop a group discussion on the links between self-esteem, confidence and health and why it is important to raise women's self-esteem in relation to health. Are women who value themselves and see themselves as equal to others more able to stand up for their rights and get their needs met?

2 Give out the handout. Either read it out loud or ask women to spend a few moments reading it on their own. End the session by asking women how they feel about the poem. Are parts of it easier to relate to their experiences than others? Why? What would be the implications for their health if they were this 'me'?

Issues raised

Women may talk about being criticised or put down and how that can affect their sense of self by contributing to a lack of confidence and leading to stress or distress in their lives (see the exercises in section 9 on criticism). You could include some gentle relaxation in the programme, or give some examples of stress management techniques. Try *Every woman's health* (see page xviii) which has sections on relaxation and stress. You could follow this exercise with one such as *TV characters* (2B), which draws similar links between self-esteem and health.

2B TV characters

EXERCISE

Purpose

To explore what we mean by high and low self-esteem and how they affect our confidence and health.

Suitable for

Large groups of women particularly. This is a light-hearted exercise and is good to use after something 'heavy'.

Materials

Flipchart paper and pens.

Method

1   Ask women to split up into pairs and identify TV characters (from, for example, *Eastenders*, *Neighbours*, and so on) who, in their opinion, have high or low self-esteem.

2   Ask women:

- How do you know these characters have high or low self-esteem?

- What do the characters say?

- How do they behave?

3   Draw up a list with the group of the adjectives they might use to describe these characters. For example:

- nervous

- good-looking

- intelligent

- lacking in confidence

- shy

- healthy emotionally and physically.

Separate these adjectives into those which indicate high or low self-esteem.

4   Now ask women to give themselves marks out of ten in relation to these attributes. Ideally, how high would participants like to be on the scale of one to ten, and why?

Discussion

1   In threes or fours, ask women to choose three positive qualities from the high self-esteem list developed earlier that they would like to have.

2   Ask women to look at each quality and discuss in which situations it would be useful. Are there any situations in which they have already used it? How would their self-esteem be improved by having this quality?

3   Bring the groups back together and ask each woman to describe her chosen qualities.

Variation

You could close the exercise here or add the following piece to it, if you have time. You could also use this part of the exercise as an 'ending' to other exercises where appropriate.

1   Ask women to settle down and make themselves

comfortable. In a calm, relaxing voice, ask them to close their eyes and to imagine a situation for a few moments, and the quality they would most like to have in that situation. Ask the group:

- What would it be like to have this quality in that situation?

- What difference would it make if you had that quality?

- How would you be different if you had that quality?

- What other qualities might change the situation again?

2 Tell the group to relax and enjoy feeling, seeing, and being these positive qualities. Ask women to visualise what the implications might be for their health if they had these qualities. Give the group three or four minutes to relax. Tell them to begin to move slowly when they are ready. Ask women to open their eyes and bring back their chosen qualities with them.

3 Go round the group for feedback on the exercise. Ask women how they feel now about the qualities they have chosen, and how they think they might be useful in the future, especially in relation to their health.

2C Haystack

E X E R C I S E

Purpose
To provide space for women to talk about and acknowledge themselves and what is important to them. To listen to others. To increase women's confidence by talking about themselves.

Suitable for
The beginning of a group or session. It was one of the most popular exercises used on the Project. It enables a group to listen and share, and quieter women in the group can be encouraged to speak up.

Materials
None. If you are running an ongoing course or have an opportunity to contact women beforehand, ask women to bring in an object that means a lot to them personally.

Method
1 Ask each woman to put a personal possession (a photograph or a bracelet, for example) into a pile in the middle of the circle and to say what it is.

2 Ask each woman to choose something that is not hers. The woman it belongs to should then tell the group:

- What is important to her about this possession.

- What it is that makes it special to her.

Discussion

When each woman has spoken about her possession, explore with the group the importance and meaning of possessions. People choose things because they are in some way a reflection of themselves. If we ourselves didn't have this quality, we wouldn't recognise it in other things. If something beautiful is special to us, it reflects the beauty inside us.

Move on to exercises such as *Me* (2D) to help women to develop their sense of self further.

2D Me

E X E R C I S E

Purpose

To encourage women to think about themselves and to get to know themselves better.

Suitable for

A group that has already begun to look at self-esteem.

Materials

A copy of handout 2B for each woman, pens.

Method

Give out the handout, and ask women to spend a few moments filling it in. Then ask them to pair up to discuss what they have written. Which were the most difficult questions to answer? The easiest? How do they feel about that?

Discussion

Bring the group back together and ask them what it was like to do the exercise. If you have enough time, end by asking each woman to read out her list assertively; otherwise, you could get each woman to read out a couple of things assertively.

Issues raised

Women may find some of the questions difficult to answer so encourage them to have a go but leave them if they are unable. Their partners might be able to help if they get stuck.

2E One hour for me

EXERCISE

Purpose

To encourage women to explore their feelings and experiences about taking time for themselves.

Suitable for

A warm-up exercise in 'down' times – after lunch, or with groups (such as mother and toddler groups) who feel guilty about taking time for themselves.

Materials

Flipchart paper and pens.

Method

Get the group to think individually about the following questions: 'If you had an hour to yourself for your health, what would you do?' Get women to brainstorm and write their answers on the flipchart. The answers might include the following.

- A bath with music
- Take a long walk
- Relax in a chair for an hour and do nothing
- Listen to music
- Window shopping
- Arrange to visit a friend without the children
- Play a relaxation tape

Variation

Give out handout 2C and ask women to fill it in.

Discussion

Follow this with a discussion (either in small groups or one group) about how women feel about doing things for themselves. Is it possible to do these things without feeling guilty or selfish? What can women do about that? You could then discuss the effects on our health when we don't take time for ourselves (depression, headaches, comfort eating, and so on).

Issues raised

- This is a very simple yet useful exercise: it often demonstrates the difficulty women have in identifying how they spend time on themselves. It also shows that women expect to have to give to others, and see time for themselves as a guilt-provoking luxury.

- Follow this session with one from *Rights and responsibilities* to enable women to look in more depth at why getting their own needs met is important.

(Many thanks to Ann Gilbert of Sandwell Social Services for material for handout 2C.)

2A I am me

In all the world there is no one else exactly like me.

Everything that comes out of me is my own because I alone choose it.

I own everything about me – my body, my feelings, my mouth, my voice, all my actions (whether they be towards others or myself).

I own my own fantasies, my dreams, my hopes, my fears. I own all my triumphs and successes, all my failures and mistakes. Because I own all of me I can get to know me very well. By doing so I can love me and be a friend to all of me.

I know there are things about me that puzzle me and other things about me which I do not know. As long as I am friendly and loving to myself I can courageously and hopefully look for solutions to the puzzles and for ways to find out more about me.

However I look and sound, whatever I do or say and whatever I think and feel at a given moment in time is me. If later some parts of how I looked, sounded, thought and felt don't fit any more, I can discard them, keep the rest and fill the space with other things which are more relevant to who I am now.

I may be able to see, hear, feel, think, say and do. I have the tools to survive and to be healthy, to be close to others, to be productive; and to make sense and order out of the world – of people and things outside of me.

I own me and therefore I can make who I am. I am me and . . .

I AM OK

2B Me

I am happiest when . . .

I feel important when . . .

I get angry when . . .

I see myself as . . .

Something I'm good at is . . .

I have always wanted to . . .

I relax by . . .

I look forward to . . .

I believe that . . .

I feel most confident when . . .

When I am healthy I am . . .

2C Things I do for myself that I enjoy

1   What are they?

2   How long is it since I did them?

3   Do I do them alone or with someone else?

4   Do they cost money?

3 How we talk to ourselves

All of us have thoughts and feelings about everything we think, feel and do. Some of these may be fleeting moments where all we say to ourselves is 'I will do that now' or 'That can wait'. But when we are depressed or feeling low mentally and physically we can often perpetuate these feelings by the things we say to ourselves – 'I shouldn't be feeling this', 'I should be able to cope' or 'I can't cope', 'People don't like me, I'm not worth bothering with'. A whole series of these 'tapes' may be running in our heads at any given moment. In some situations, what we say to ourselves may be the major factor stopping us from standing our ground and asserting ourselves effectively.

The following exercises give women an opportunity to explore how what we say to ourselves affects our behaviour. Handout 3A gives some specific examples of how this might happen. Raising awareness of this can often:

- help women to see that they are not the only ones who have unvoiced fears about things;

- enable women to develop different ways of thinking in the future.

3A How we talk to ourselves

EXERCISE

Purpose
To get participants to look at how their thoughts and feelings can influence their assertive and non-assertive behaviour in relation to their health.

Suitable for
Any group of women. It is particularly good to use with older women, some of whom find having to go for smear tests and breast examinations, for instance, difficult and perhaps alarming. This exercise enables such women to voice their fears and provides a forum for reassurance. If you are running this type of group, or think these issues may come up, gather as much information as you can about the issues to give out to women. Contact your local health education/promotion unit for details of how to get leaflets, etc.

Materials

A copy of handout 3A for each woman. (Or the first page of the handout, with a drawing of each face on a large sheet of paper.)

Method

1   Using both the handout and the faces, begin by outlining what talking to ourselves and 'tapes' are about.

2   Ask women to pair up and think of a situation in which they feel confident. They should then discuss the situation with their partners, asking themselves the following questions.

   ● What do I say to myself in the situation?

   ● How do I feel physically?

   ● What happens as a result?

3   Ask participants to think of a situation where they don't feel confident. Get them to ask themselves the same questions as above.

4   Ask women to look at the situation in which they lack confidence. Get them to discuss the following with their partners.

   ● How could I be more assertive and positive about myself in this situation?

   ● How could I make myself feel differently (e.g., positive 'tape', taking more time, breathing deeply)?

   ● How could I behave differently in the future (assertively, positively, confidently)?

5   Finally, ask women to run through the situation in which they lack confidence with their partner, using positive 'tapes'.

Discussion

1   Bring the group back together and ask women to feed back their situations and the 'tapes' they will try to use in the future.

2   End the exercise by asking women to relax and close their eyes. Gently ask them to imagine playing themselves a positive 'tape' in the future. You could use *I am me* (handout 2A) to end the session on a confidence-enhancing note.

Variation

1   After discussing the handout and the faces women could draw their own pictures of themselves and add words or phrases that go with their positive and negative 'tapes'. These could then be discussed in pairs.

2   You could also use *The confidence tree* (page 26). After discussing the handout and faces, ask women to look at it and identify what they think each person on the tree is saying to herself at that moment. The good mixture of positive and negative images on the tree will promote discussion. This is a good way of getting the message of 'tapes' across if you have only a short time.

3B Feeling good about ourselves

EXERCISE

Purpose

To encourage women to look at being positive about themselves: hearing the positive things people say about them and believing them.

Suitable for

Groups that prefer talking, since it is mostly discussion based. Remember that women may not be used to being positive about themselves, and may need to be encouraged to keep at it when trying to find good things to say about themselves.

Materials

A copy of handout 3B for each woman.

Method

1   As a group, discuss the following questions:

   • Do we believe we can feel good about ourselves?

   • How do we react when somebody says, 'I like the way you look today'?

   • What kinds of things make us feel good about ourselves?

2   Ask women to fill in the handout before the next session. (Encourage them to think of specific things that might benefit their general health.)

3   Point out that ordinary, everyday things that make us feel good are important to note – newly washed or styled hair; reading a book or article that has a good effect on us;

someone paying us a compliment; saving a half-dead plant; taking the trouble to visit someone lonely, and so on.

Discussion

- End the session by asking each woman to think of at least one positive thing she will do for herself before the next session.

- Ensure that discussion time is built in to the next session so that participants can feed back their experiences of filling out the handout.

Issues raised

This kind of exercise could raise issues about what contributes to women's low self-esteem (dealing with physical or emotional abuse; unrealistic expectations about women's roles as mothers, partners, lovers, daughters, employees, and so on). It could also be linked with how low self-esteem can affect women's ability to assert themselves in relation to their health.

3A How we talk to ourselves

- Being assertive is not just about how we deal with other people. Another important element is how we talk to ourselves.

- We are always telling ourselves stories and making images about how things will be if we do this or that. These patterns of thinking then influence our behaviour.

- Below are examples of ways we talk to ourselves, and the influence this can have on outcomes.

Situation A: deciding whether to ask the GP what exactly he or she means by Candida.

Negative tape: he or she will think I am being a nuisance, and I should know what it means anyway.

Consequence: don't ask, then feel worse afterwards. Risk worsening the infection because of the worry and stress of not knowing.

Situation B: deciding whether to ask for a plastic speculum instead of a cold metal one for this smear test.

Negative tape: the metal one is ready and I would be holding up other patients by asking. They probably wouldn't give me one anyway.

Consequence: suffer a cold metal speculum! And feel bad about not having said anything.

Situation C: deciding whether to ask for a second opinion on a medical matter.

Positive tape: this is my body and I have the right to ensure that I explore all the options that might be available to me.

Consequence: feel good about asserting yourself and feel more in control of your body and what happens to it.

As you can see from the first two examples, we can often be our own worst enemies, sabotaging possible positive outcomes by negative thoughts.

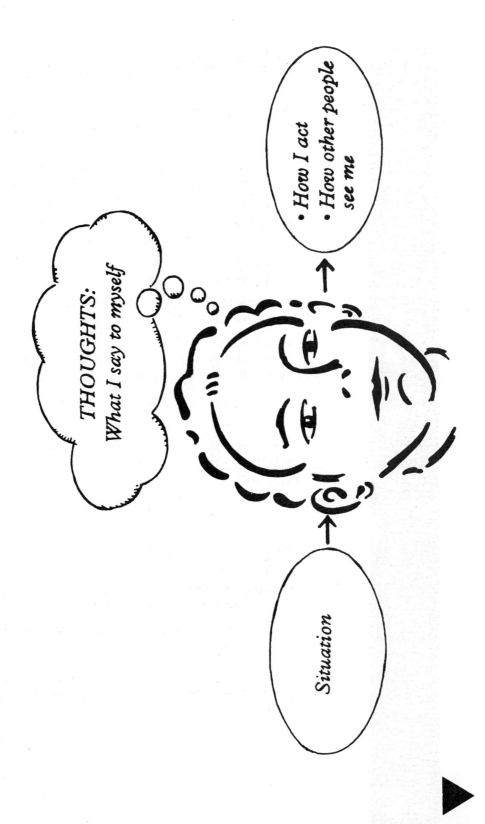

THOUGHTS:
What I say to myself

• How I act
• How other people see me

Situation

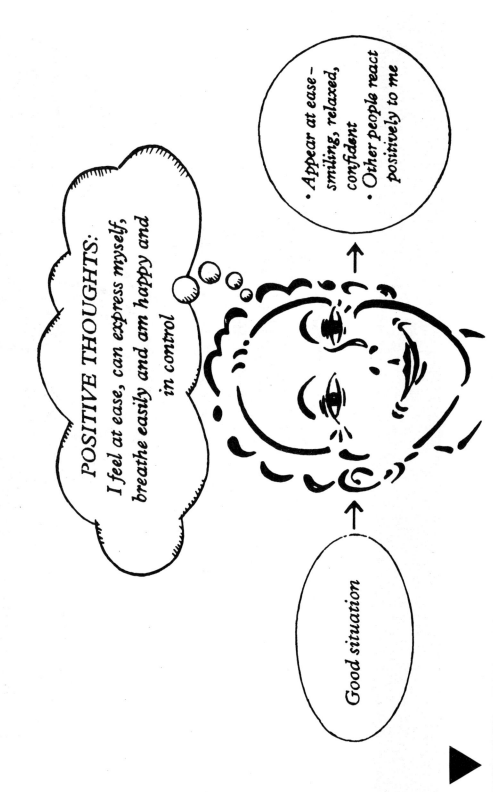

POSITIVE THOUGHTS:
I feel at ease, can express myself, breathe easily and am happy and in control

- Appear at ease – smiling, relaxed, confident
- Other people react positively to me

Good situation

Handout 3A

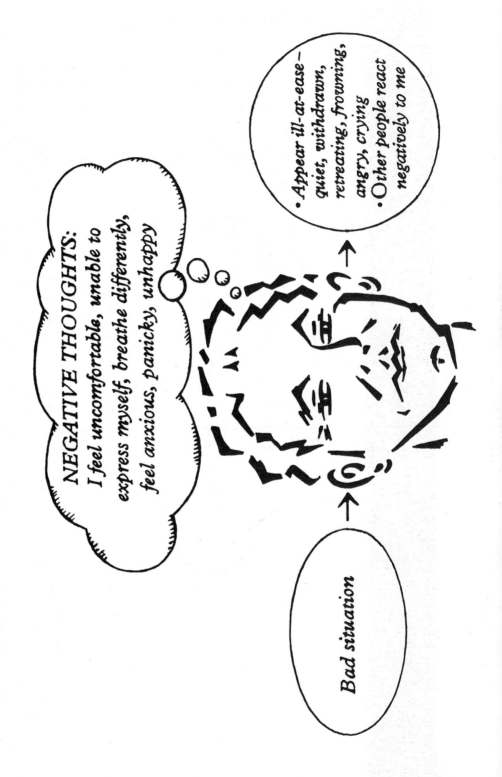

3B Thinking positively

On each day of the week write something positive about yourself. You could ask yourself, for example:

- What do I like about myself today?
- What have I achieved today?
- Did I handle a particular situation well?

DAY 1

DAY 2

DAY 3

DAY 4

DAY 5

DAY 6

DAY 7

4 How we see ourselves

Exploring how women see themselves in relation to others' expectations of them highlights a number of issues.

Hardly anyone has the classic model's body, and yet women are encouraged to aspire to it through the media. Alongside this are the assumptions people make about us (and those we make about others) on the basis of the way we look, the colour of our skin or hair; as well as on the basis of our roles as mothers, lovers, partners, daughters and so on. These assumptions rarely match how we feel about ourselves inside.

Enabling women to explore their own self-images and encouraging and supporting them in developing a healthy and confident image can considerably enhance their ability to be assertively healthy. Believing fully in who and what we are and having a strong sense of our own identity is a big step towards a healthier lifestyle.

Case study: self-image and sex-role stereotyping

The following work was undertaken with a group of young women from various youth clubs at a residential weekend which looked at assertiveness and health.

The original intention was to look at self-image and sex-role stereotyping with the whole group. However, after witnessing situations and encounters when they and the young women went out on the Saturday evening, the facilitators decided to change the programme.

They decided to use the first half of Sunday morning to set up a role-play 're-run' of this fairly typical Saturday night out, and to encourage the participants to develop the scenario for themselves. The intention was to stop them at various points and ask them questions about their thoughts, feelings and (if need be) how they could be more assertive and perhaps change the course of events.

During the exercise issues of harassment (both male- and female-initiated), peer pressure, misinformation and sex-role expectations were explored. Assertiveness techniques were rehearsed, and the possible consequences of some of their actions were looked at.

The group facilitators felt the scenario provided ideal material for putting assertiveness into practice in a real situation for the group. Neither of the facilitators had used this method before, though they had used role play. It proved to be a dynamic (as well as innovative) experience for the group.

This is a valuable way of working with young people, and could be used in a variety of situations. It is active, fun, developmental and real for them – satisfying all the important educational considerations.

We do recommend, however, that facilitators practise using this method before launching themselves into it with a group or course. One of the difficulties was knowing the right moment to intervene. Facilitators also need to be clear about whether to let the exercise take its own course or to direct it in particular ways towards particular issues.

This way of working requires a lot of skill and can be difficult to keep on track. Nevertheless, it was found to be very worthwhile and interesting and certainly worth developing.

4A Images of women

EXERCISE

Purpose

To explore the messages that magazines in particular and the media in general send out about women and stereotypes.

Suitable for

- This exercise uses collage and is a straightforward and active group exercise. It is a great way of creating starting points for discussion on health and assertiveness and requires very little literacy skill because it uses mostly visual images. Any reading or writing that is required can be shared by the group. It can be used at any stage and is ideal as a 'gelling' exercise for a group once ground rules have been established.

- It is suitable for all ages, but may particularly stimulate young women. If women have impaired sight you could also use tapes of radio programmes or good sound-quality videos of adverts on TV. You could then look at how voiceovers and commentaries portray women (usually using male voices to sell us something!).

Materials

You need to collect, probably for some time in advance, magazines containing articles, photographs or drawings of women. Try to ensure that there is a wide variety of magazines – include ones such as *Everywoman*, the *Pink Paper* (or other lesbian or gay publications) and any black and minority ethnic publications (*Essence*, *Pride*) you can find. You will also need scissors and glue, and large sheets of paper.

Method

1   To set the scene, begin with a short discussion on how women are portrayed in the media.

2   Divide the group into threes or fours and give each group a selection of magazines. Ask each to use the images and words they find in the magazines to produce a collage depicting how they themselves and others perceive women in relation to sexual health and health in general. Ask them to try and depict all women – with and without disabilities, young, older, of different sizes, sexualities, races and communities, happy, sad, working, as mothers, friends, and so on.

Variation

Give each group a special topic – women and romance; women and motherhood, and so on.

Discussion

1   Discuss as a group the main images in each of the collages. Get women to describe what thoughts and feelings doing the exercise has inspired. What are the limitations of images of women in the media? What do the collages say about women's health and how we should look and feel as opposed to how we really do?

2   Develop the discussion by asking women to look at the collages and identify women by age, disability and so on. Are any of the pictures of lesbians? What assumptions do we make on the basis of appearance? If there are no black or minority ethnic women, women with disabilities, and so on, bring this up and explore why.

Issues raised

When this exercise was undertaken on the Project with a group of young women with learning difficulties it began to raise awareness about how women are seen and what they *should* and *could* be doing in their lives. It was evident from the group's work that very young women often have strongly stereotypical views of what a woman does and how she should look. The workers involved felt that if attitudes towards women are to change, girls' expectations of their own development need to be challenged, and they need to be encouraged to explore different roles from the ones normally presented to them – as passive, carers, and so on.

4B Drawing our own images of ourselves

E X E R C I S E

Purpose

- To encourage participants to think about how they see themselves.
- To explore the links between self-image and health.

Suitable for

Using after *Images of women* (4A), so you move from looking at images of women in general to looking at women's perceptions of themselves.

Materials

Flipchart paper (one sheet for each woman) and lots of different coloured pens in different sizes.

Method

1   Ask each woman to have a go at drawing herself, in any way she likes – as a stick figure, in parts, etc. Explain that the purpose is not to produce works of art but to think about how we see ourselves.

2   Get women to discuss, in pairs or threes, how it felt to draw their image.

3   Still in the pairs or threes, ask participants to discuss what their drawing says about them. Do the others agree? Are there anxieties shared by all the women in the group?

Discussion

In the main group draw out the common issues that came up in the small groups. (If you have done the *Images of women* collages, you could look at these again and discuss the role these representations have in shaping women's images of themselves.) What are the health implications of women feeling the way they do about themselves? Ask women what they could do to lessen the anxieties they have about themselves, and finish with each woman identifying one anxiety and one thing she could do to lessen its effect on her.

4C The me I like and the me I don't like

EXERCISE

Purpose

To enable women to discuss and explore difficulties in being positive about themselves.

Suitable for

Giving women an opportunity to 'balance' their negative and positive thoughts about themselves. Can be used after discussions on women's roles and how they feel about them, or as a prelude to exercises on criticism and/or compliments. Good for groups with low literacy or groups who are fed up with flipchart and pens!

Materials

A4 paper and pens, if women want to make lists.

Method

1   Ask participants to list three things they don't like about themselves ('I have big feet' . . .). Get them to pair up and discuss them with a partner. Taking turns, the pair should look at one thing at a time, challenging each other's statements if they wish to, or supporting other positive aspects ('Have you? They don't look very big to me'; or 'Well, yes, perhaps they are. However, those shoes you're wearing look great.')

2   Ask participants to list three things they like about themselves and discuss them with a partner ('I like my sense of humour'). This can be a bit harder, and can produce some humour and groans, but it also provides the opportunity to discuss why women find it difficult to be positive about themselves.

Variation

If you are running a group that meets regularly or you have an opportunity to meet the group before the session, ask women to bring an object that represents something positive about themselves to the session (a photo, perfume, a book, for example). This can be a good way of 'opening up' women to thinking about being positive about themselves. Ask each woman to show her object and to explain why and how it represents her. Ensure that everything they say remains positive and gently challenge any negative things that may creep in.

Discussion

In the main group, explain that having a positive attitude to ourselves and what we do is vital if we are to be healthy and lead full lives. One thing we can take control of is our thoughts about ourselves. Acknowledging the things we don't like about ourselves is the first step to changing them. Balancing them out with things we feel positive about helps us to see ourselves more clearly. End the session by asking each woman to say something that she feels good about in herself.

4D Giving and receiving compliments

E X E R C I S E

Purpose

To encourage women to practise giving and receiving compliments as a way of nurturing their emotional health.

Suitable for

Groups who have been working together for a while and/or who know each other well and feel safe. (Although this is not intended as an in-depth session.) Because this exercise asks women to compliment each other, make sure that they do not concentrate on appearance alone. In a society that rates women mainly on their appearance and attractiveness it is important to value women's inner qualities and strengths.

Materials

None.

Method

1 Begin by developing a discussion about what it is like to pay compliments to other people and the difficulties that might be involved if the other person is suspicious of your motives, thinks you are 'after something', and so on. It is often just as difficult to accept the positive things that are said about us – perhaps 'putting down' the other person, or shrugging off the remark with something like, 'Oh, this old thing?', or 'Do you really think that?'

2 Ask participants to help arrange chairs into two circles, one facing out and the other facing inwards, so that each woman has a partner.

3 Ask each woman to think of something nice to say to her partner, and then say it. Suggest that women don't spend too much time thinking of what to say – compliments are often spontaneous reactions.

4   Ask the women in pairs to think of how they would react
     if someone said that to them – be positive, but keep it
     simple.

5   Ask women to tell their partner what they like about her,
     wait for her response, and then ask the outside circle to
     move round two spaces and repeat. Do this as many times
     as the group feels comfortable with. Finally, split them into
     two groups and ask them to discuss what it felt like to give
     the compliments and what it felt like to receive them.

Discussion

1   How did women feel about having to think of
     compliments? Was it easier with some women than others?
     Were they afraid that it might be misinterpreted? What
     was it like to be complimented? Was their initial reaction to
     dismiss it? Ask each woman to identify one of the
     compliments she was given and how she felt about it.

2   End the session with a group discussion on giving and
     receiving compliments.

5 Communicating with others

Body language and non-verbal communication are another area vital to assertiveness. Being assertive involves much more than learning what the 'right' verbal response might be in any given situation. Our entire body can help us to assert ourselves positively. Attempts to manage a situation may fail even if the words are exactly right, if what come across is uncertainty, self-doubt or hostility.

We don't have to adopt a whole new set of postures or ways of behaving in order to become more successful at matching what we say with how we feel about saying it. Rather, we need to look at how we can unlearn the things that prevent us from acting assertively, replacing them with postures and behaviours more 'in tune' with what we are doing.

The following exercises can help women identify new ways of linking what they feel and what they do.

5A Body language and non-verbal communication

E X E R C I S E

Purpose
To enable women to look at what 'standing our ground' can mean on both a physical and emotional level.

Suitable for
Linking exercises that look at how women feel about assertiveness and health with ones (such as *Charades*, 5B) which aim to show the importance of non-verbal communication in assertive behaviour. This exercise requires women to stand up for a short time, so ensure before you start that this is possible.

Materials
None.

Method
1   Ask the group to look around at everyone in the room. What is their body language telling you?

2   Ask women to stand up and just think about a situation where they would like to assert themselves. (They don't have to say what the situation is, just think about it.)

3   Ask the group what they notice about other women in the group now. Do they stand with their weight more on one foot, for example? (This might mean that they are physically unbalanced when trying to deal with something difficult.)

4   Now ask women to stand on both feet with their weight equally distributed and their bodies as upright as possible. Ask what feels different and how it might affect their chosen situation if they were to stand like this.

Discussion

1   Ask women to sit down. Has the preceding exercise enabled them to feel more assertive? If we want to be heard saying something we need to stand our ground physically as well as mentally – giving out much more powerful messages. Discuss how women in wheelchairs or women who are unable to stand upright may be able to assert themselves on a physical level. Read out the success story (page 80) and encourage women to share any successes of their own.

2   Ask each woman to tell one other person about one situation over the next week where she might be able to use body language to be more assertive. If this is a course where the group will come back together, make sure that you leave enough time at the beginning of the next session to feed back these situations.

Issues raised

●   In discussions on body language, it is also important to introduce the concept of 'power games' that people play. For example, women have found it useful to be made aware of the deliberate positioning of office furniture – in a GP's surgery, in a bank, in a head-teacher's office and at interviews – to give those in charge of the arrangement control of the situation.

●   While in many situations we cannot do anything to change the layout of the room, being aware of it gives us power. We feel less 'put down' or intimidated when we are aware of what is happening in these unspoken games.

Success story

One woman made use of the information on 'power games' in a recent visit to a consultant. The consultant was sitting behind a large desk, across the room from her (low-level) chair. Quickly assessing the situation, she picked up the chair, moved it up to the desk, and leaned on the edge of the desk.

While she did not achieve what she wanted from the consultation, she left feeling good about herself – she had been in control, and had been aware of the 'power games' being played. A potentially demoralising situation had become only a disappointment, in that she didn't achieve the result she wanted, but she was able to recognise what was happening in the situation.

5B Charades

EXERCISE

Purpose

- To draw participants' attention to different aspects of non-verbal communication.

- To provide participants with an opportunity to express and identify non-verbal attitudes and feelings.

Suitable for

Introducing the importance of matching our non-verbal actions to our verbal actions. An enjoyable and fun way of teaching non-verbal communication.

Materials

Separate pieces of paper. Write a range of attitudes and feelings on the pieces of paper: shy, confident, angry, patronising, happy, unsure, critical, sad, surprised, confused, unhappy, questioning, and so on. Underneath each one write, 'I don't know what to say'.

Method

1 Ask each member of the group to select one of the pieces of paper you have prepared and say the sentence in the manner described. The rest of the group then has to guess the attitude or feeling expressed.

2 Get the group to brainstorm the kind of clues they got – tone of voice, hand gestures, and so on.

Discussion

1 Ask the group how it felt to say the sentences in the manner described. Then ask how it felt to guess the attitude or feeling. Was it easy or difficult?

2 Discuss with the group the point of the exercise: that it's often not what is said that's important but *how* it is said. Learning how to read the feeling or attitude behind what people say and then responding to that is a very important communication skill.

Issues raised

Participants may find this exercise difficult to get into although once they do, it powerfully reinforces the importance of verbal and non-verbal communication.

5C Getting what we want and feeling confident

EXERCISE

Purpose

To stimulate discussion and clarify particular areas related to health where women experience difficulty trying to be assertive.

Suitable for

Providing a lot of useful material for discussion. Use it before exercises about saying no or dealing with criticism, so that women have identified situations that are 'real' to them. Use the handout as a guide and add other questions appropriate to this group.

Materials

Either a copy of handout 5A for each woman, or flipchart paper with the questions written on it.

Method

Ask women to look at each question on the handout and discuss their responses with the person next to them. Ask them also to rank their responses in terms of which situations would be easier to deal with assertively and why, and which would be more difficult and why.

Discussion

1 Ask women to feed back what it was like to go through the list. Is it easier, for instance, to be more assertive with

strangers than with friends or people close to you? If so, why? Is it easier to deal with health issues on behalf of other people than on your own behalf?

2   End the discussion by asking women to state one thing they have become more aware of by doing the exercise. Ask them to bear in mind the situations they have identified, to use in future sessions.

5D Becoming more healthy and assertive

E X E R C I S E

Purpose

To explore potential blocks women may have about being more assertive in relation to their health.

Suitable for

Groups of women who may feel they have too much to lose if they become more assertive. This exercise enables them to discuss their fears about asserting themselves. Facilitators can then build on this to work on issues that women feel they may safely be able to do something tangible about. This exercise should be done following a basic introduction to assertive, aggressive and passive behaviour types, such as exercise 1F.

Materials

Paper and pens. A copy of handout 5B for each woman.

Method

1   Ask participants to make a list of situations relating to their health in which they need to become more confident – situations where the outcome needs to be under their control. Use prompt list 1 if the group finds it hard to identify situations. Ask them then to number their list in order of priority, with the least difficult first.

2   Ask the women to form groups of three and tell each other how they behave now in these situations – passively, aggressively, manipulatively or defensively – beginning with their first situation. What are they telling themselves at the time? What might the implications be for their health in both the short and the long term? (Use prompt list 2 at this point, if necessary.) Repeat with the rest of the situations.

3   Ask women, still in small groups, to write or discuss possible assertive responses to these situations. Ask them to focus particularly on what they would be telling

themselves in the situation which would be different from
before. (Use prompt list 3.)

4   Now ask women to try out the different responses. This is
best done in threes, with one person acting as an observer,
one as herself and one as the other person involved in the
situation. Encourage women to help each other come up
with different ways of dealing with the situations, and
include an emphasis on body language when women are
practising the responses.

Discussion

1   Feed back what happened when women tried out their
new responses and how they feel about them. What would
be the implications for their short- and long-term health if
they did things this way?

2   End the session by asking each woman to state one
situation she has identified and one way of changing it for
the better. If the group will be meeting again, ask women
to make a note of one situation they have handled
assertively and one that they have not before the time you
next meet. Begin the next session with feedback on this
and ask them what the experiences felt like and how they
might handle them in the future.

Issues raised

●   This exercise could lead to discussions on how far women
might feel able to go in terms of assertiveness. Asking
questions such as 'What would happen if you did assert
yourself?' may elicit how (like one group in the Project)
they feel they can only do so much work on changing their
behaviour. They may be anxious that their partners will
leave them, or their friends or families will accuse them of
not being 'nice', or health workers will behave as though
they are being difficult. Facilitators should see this as a very
positive stage in the group's life. People need to be
encouraged to get over these blocks – and these issues
often only come out when women start to see, or feel, that
they could change if they wanted to.

●   The difficulties of asserting ourselves when dealing with
hierarchical organisations or situations may come up – for
example, being scared to ask a doctor for clarification or
further information, finding it even more difficult to ask a
consultant, but easy to ask a nurse.

5A What do you do?

1 When a friend asks you to have another drink and you don't want one, can you refuse?

2 If you do not understand what your doctor is telling you, can you insist that he or she explains?

3 Are you able to tell your partner (if you have one) what you want or don't want sexually or emotionally?

4 When you need help, is it easy for you to ask others to give it to you?

5 Do you feel confident about dealing assertively with health professionals about your own health? And about others' health (your children, parents, and so on)?

6 If you feel hurt by something a friend has said or done, can you tell him or her how you feel?

5B Becoming more healthy and assertive

Prompt list 1

Dealing with legal people

Dealing with court officials

Dealing with doctors about personal issues

Talking to health visitors

Giving constructive criticism at work

Having to say 'I don't agree' in small groups of people

Dealing with racism/sexism/ageism/heterosexism, and so on

Refusing a drink

Dealing with sexual advances or remarks

Dealing with sexual harassment in interviews

Dealing with family conflicts

Responding to being ignored by shopkeepers

Choosing a contraceptive with my partner

Prompt list 2

I feel:

- sick
- powerless
- out of control
- inadequate
- disloyal
- quiet
- self-critical
- angry

- panicked
- too talkative
- annoyed

Prompt list 3

I am:

- able to challenge this situation
- in control
- able to ask the 'right' questions
- sensible
- sticking to my point of view confidently
- getting what I want from the situation
- calm, relaxed and assertive

6 Health and sexual health

This section deals specifically with health, sexual health and assertiveness. Sharing experiences in groups can often give women the confidence to do things they might otherwise have backed away from – going to the doctor about a lump, asserting themselves with a family member who is causing them some distress, challenging racist or ageist statements, and so on.

This group of exercises moves from looking at health and assertiveness generally, to negotiating sexual relationships and specific sexual health issues.

6A Health – what is it?

EXERCISE

Purpose
To enable women to review their experiences of behaving assertively and how they feel physically and emotionally when they do so. The exercise also brings up how they feel when they don't behave assertively.

Suitable for
Using with young women to get them thinking about health on a broad level.

Materials
Flipchart, paper and pens. For the variation: a copy of handout 6A for each woman.

Method
1 Begin the exercise by saying that being healthy can also mean feeling confident and being able to take decisions that affect our physical, emotional and sexual lives. To be able to assert ourselves convincingly we need to feel good about ourselves and 'value a self worth asserting'.

2 Get the whole group to discuss what is meant by physical and emotional health.

3 Then divide the group into two.

Group one – brainstorm onto flipchart paper what it is like to be physically unhealthy: aches and pains, tired, pale, overweight/underweight, and so on.

Group two – brainstorm onto flipchart paper what it is like to be emotionally unhealthy: depressed, under stress, and so on.

4 Get the groups to feed back to each other on their ideas.

Variation

1 Give out copies of handout 6A and ask women to fill it in for themselves. Divide the group into two and ask each group to discuss what they have written.

2 Ask each group to come up with a definition of health.

3 Bring the groups back together and feed back definitions.

Discussion

Promote discussion around the definitions. Are they positive or negative? Do women in the group experience physical and emotional 'unhealth'? How do they deal with it?

End the session by offering information on where to seek further help (friendship, support and/or professional support and advice) if required (see *Resources* section). Follow or add to this session with exercises on relaxation and ways of managing stress.

Issues raised

When this exercise was used with women aged 14–17 in the Project, a lot of information was shared about experiences of depression, stress and self-harm – a whole range of emotional health issues. Facilitators were concerned about some group members' experiences and spent a lot of time encouraging group members to support each other. Ground rules that had been set at the beginning came into their own here. It was essential that the confidentiality which had been agreed meant that trust was not broken in the group.

(Many thanks to Kath Winn of Clwyd Health Promotion Unit for providing the project with this handout.)

6B What affects your health?

E X E R C I S E

Purpose

To enable women to explore what affects their health.

Suitable for

All groups.

Materials

A copy of handout 6B for each woman, pens.

Method

This exercise can be done:

- individually;

- individually, followed by general feedback;

- as a group, putting together ideas about what influences health.

Give out the handouts. Tell women that they are at the centre of the rings and that they should fill in the other rings as follows:

- **In the inner ring**, write down personal things that affect your health – e.g. family, home, work, food, attitudes, etc.

- **In the second ring**, write down things that affect your health within your immediate social and physical environment – friends, colleagues, locality, community, facilities and services, etc.

- **In the outer ring**, write down things that affect your health which are connected to your wider social, cultural, physical, religious and political environment – legislation, environmental issues, etc.

Discussion

1 Ask the group to consider the following questions:

- How do these things influence your health – positively or negatively?

- Which things do you think are the most important?

- Are there things that you have not identified for yourself, but which may be important for other people?

2 Close by asking women how it felt to do the exercise and to note any points that may be useful to them in the future.

Issues raised

This type of exercise can reveal that women's self-esteem, and consequently their health, can suffer because of factors they cannot control – having to live in poor accommodation, perhaps. Support needs to be given to help women to explore what, if anything, can be done to help their situation. When preparing sessions like this, bear in mind that you will need to know (by networking and maintaining contact with other agencies) when to refer women for help.

6C Being healthy

E X E R C I S E

Purpose

To enable participants to look at their own health and what is stopping them from being healthy. To develop participants' understanding that health is affected by much wider influences than notions of illness (for example, lack of money, transport, childcare, lack of self-confidence etc.).

Suitable for

All groups.

Materials

A copy of handout 6C for each woman, pens.

Method

Ask participants to draw, write on or talk through the handout with a partner, then discuss with each other the issues that arise.

Variation

If the group has difficulty writing things down, you could adapt the exercise in one of the following ways:

1   Whoever finds it most easy to write can put down what everybody brainstorms under the two headings.

2   Run the exercise as a group discussion.

Discussion

Finish with a feedback session with the whole group sharing what has come up as a result of the exercise. These very simple exercises are often the ones that promote the most thinking and learning for participants.

6D Asking for what I want

E X E R C I S E

Purpose

To give women an opportunity to explore what they want in relation to health. How easy or difficult is it to ask for what they want?

Suitable for

An informal group or one with a limited amount of discussion time.

Materials

A copy of handout 6D for each woman.

Method

Give out copies of the handout. Ask women to think about, and discuss in pairs, these and other situations where they need to ask for what they want.

All of these situations are associated with problems which are usually due to external pressures and expectations. Women have to be able to stick with their decisions, despite pressure which may be intense.

Acting assertively can be tiring sometimes so explain to the group the importance of being clear within their own minds about what they do and don't want and to see it as 'teaching' people about what they want.

6E Good and bad experiences with health professionals

E X E R C I S E

Purpose

To encourage women to discuss their experiences of dealing with health professionals, and to explore both positive and negative experiences.

Suitable for

All groups of women. However, it can be particularly useful with groups of NHS/health workers themselves, to help them understand, through their own experiences, what it might be like for a patient or client to experience health services in both positive and negative ways.

Materials

Flipchart paper and pens.

Method

1   Ask the group what makes a difficult or bad experience with a health professional (doctor, nurse, health visitor, consultant, psychologist, etc.). Get them either to think about this on their own, or discuss it with a partner. Then ask them to feed back what they have come up with and write it up on the flipchart.

Things that might come up.

- Decisions being made for you!
- They don't know who you are
- Feeling like a third party
- Budgets more important than people
- Lack of a holistic approach to treatment
- Being expected to be a 'good' patient
- Assumptions about needs
- They don't look at you

- Disapproval and prejudice
- Lack of care
- Feeling 'flattened'
- Treatment being continued even if it hurts
- Power – theirs over you

2   Ask the group what makes a good experience with a health
    professional. Again, get them to work on this alone or in
    pairs for a few minutes, then chart the responses on
    another piece of paper.

    Things that might come up.

    - When the professionals recognise who your body
      belongs to
    - Being able to read through what you are signing
    - Being able to be empowered
    - 'Human' receptionists
    - Non-judgemental attitudes
    - Dealing with the whole patient – rather than just
      treating obvious symptoms
    - Being able to challenge bad practice without being seen
      negatively
    - Up-to-date and alternative health care choices available
      as locally as possible

Discussion

Discuss with the group how they react in each of these
situations – assertively or unassertively? In order to keep the
group focused on the issue, you could bring the discussion
round to assertiveness by asking:

- What might you do differently next time?
- How could you phrase a question to get the response you
  want?
- What do/did you want in this situation?
- What was it about the good situations that helped to
  improve things?
- How could you transfer the learning from the good
  situations to the bad ones?

Add other 'open' questions to this list from your own
experience.

Issues raised

Problems arising from this type of exercise are likely to be very real for women. Although you need to allow sufficient time for women to express their problems, it is important to ensure that the group does not become dominated by one person's issues. This exercise is best done in small groups (no more than 12) so that you are better able to 'pace' the group.

6F Sexuality and sensuality - what do they mean?

EXERCISE

Purpose

To encourage women to explore the meaning of sexuality and sensuality.

Suitable for

Using as a fun way of bringing up issues women may never have openly explored before. Do stress that it is not an art competition: some people find having to draw a complete nightmare! You could provide ready-drawn outlines as an alternative to asking the women to draw them if you think this might be a problem.

Materials

- Pictures of women's bodies cut out of magazines. Ensure that they are representative of all women in respect of age, ethnicity, disability, sexuality and so on, and that there is a range of shapes and sizes. Use publications like *Everywoman*, as well as mass-market women's magazines, in order to avoid portraying only the 'model' ideal of attractiveness.

- Flipchart paper and different-coloured pens. Ready-drawn outlines of women's bodies (optional). Definitions (dictionary or other) of sexuality and sensuality.

Method

1 Begin by giving some dictionary definitions of sexuality (broadly, to do with sex or the sexes) and sensuality (broadly, about the senses), and explain that the purpose of the session is to explore these.

2 Ask women in threes and fours to discuss the pictures and say whether the images are 'sexual' or 'sensual'.

3 Bring the groups back together and ask them to show one 'sexual' and one 'sensual' picture they came up with and to explain why they chose them.

4   Ask women to go back into their groups. Give each group one large sheet of paper and some pens (or ready-drawn bodies).

5   Ask each group to choose someone to draw an outline of a female body (if not using ready-drawn ones) and then colour in what they feel to be the sexual and sensual parts (using different-coloured pens). Each person in the group could have a pen and colour a part in turn to enable all participants to be involved.

Note: In order to get an instant response, ask participants to do the exercise in silence for a couple of minutes and then to discuss what they have come up with for a few minutes in their groups.

Discussion

1   Place the drawings from each group on the wall and begin a discussion on:

   - Who has defined these areas as sexual or sensual?

   - Are these really sexual and sensual areas in our experience?

   - Are there differences between what we regard as sexual and sensual? If so, what do we mean by each of these words?

   - Is the whole body sensual?

   - What other parts of ourselves do we feel are sexual or sensual?

2   Invite participants to return to their drawings and add anything they want – maybe changing which parts are sensual or sexual.

3   You could extend the discussion by asking participants to think about any of the following:

   - Other women's sexuality and sensuality (taboos about women touching each other are often less than those between men).

   - In what ways do we touch a friend differently from a lover?

   - Do we have the freedom to express ourselves through touching and hugging parents, children, brothers, sisters and friends, or are we discouraged from this for social or cultural reasons?

   - Are women conditioned to feel negatively or positively about the female body (stereotypes of women's bodies as erotic or highly sexed, or the negative use of words such as 'seductive')?

- What kinds of words are commonly used for each part of women's bodies, or as descriptions of women? How do women feel about, for example, the amount of words that denote food of some kind – 'crumpet', 'tart' and so on?

Issued raised

Issues raised in discussion may include the role body language plays in sensuality or sexuality, or how the portrayal of women in the media encourages us to see only some parts of our bodies as sexual and others as sensual.

6G What sexual health means to me

E X E R C I S E

Purpose

To introduce the subject of sexual health.

Suitable for

Starting to talk about sexual health and assertiveness. It introduces these issues in a relaxed way.

Materials

A basket with a collection of items relating to women's sexual health. It might contain:

- Plastic speculum
- Coil or cap
- Condom
- Vibrator
- Spermicidal cream
- Skin cream
- Prescription
- Massage oil
- Sexy knickers or nightdress
- Dental dam (oral shield)
- Pelvic model (if you are able to get one)

- Contraceptive pills
- Homoeopathic medicine for pre-menstrual syndrome
- Tampons
- Hair colouring
- Sexy book
- Female condom
- Lubricant

Be as innovative as possible when putting your basket together. Try to find items that you know will provoke discussion amongst women. Get in touch with your local family planning clinic and ask if they can let you have supplies of condoms and so on. You could also ask women to bring in their own items.

Method

Get women to sit in a circle, pass the basket around and ask each woman to take an item – preferably something they recognise or something they are interested in. What does it mean to them in relation to their sexual health? (Some may never have held a speculum in their hands before, or may not know that plastic ones are available.)

Discussion

Encourage the group to discuss the objects and their relevance to sexual health. Who do women feel their bodies belong to when they are unwell, in need of treatment, talking about what kind of sex they want, or finding suitable contraception? How might assertiveness help them gain control of their bodies?

Issues raised

Some women may feel embarrassed or offended, or have difficulty in accepting or finding relevant some of the items. (Some women may not have any choice in the contraception they use because their partner or religion demands they use a certain type; as lesbians, some women may not use contraception, and so on.) It is important to be aware of these issues and to be sensitive to the needs of the group when planning exercises of this kind.

6H Sexual health and assertiveness

EXERCISE

Purpose

To encourage women to explore how assertiveness affects both their general and their sexual health.

Suitable for

Groups who have already done some work on defining and understanding assertiveness.

Materials

Flipchart paper and pens.

Method

1   Divide women up into small groups. Give each group a piece of flipchart paper and some pens and ask them to write down any answers to the question, 'How would being more assertive affect my health?'

2   Ask them to feed back in one group what they came up with. Women in the Project came up with the following answers.

   ● I would be able to ask questions and ask people to explain if I didn't understand

   ● I could find out about my body

   ● I wouldn't feel guilty or vulnerable

   ● I wouldn't accept something I wasn't happy with

   ● People would believe me when I said no

   ● I would be able to say what I wanted

   ● I would know my rights, and ask for more information

   Do women find this list helpful? What was it like thinking about the original question?

3   Ask women to go back into the smaller groups and to brainstorm the question, 'What is sexual health?'

4   Get the smaller groups to feed back into the main group. Women in the Project came up with the following answers.

   ● Safer sex

   ● Breast care

   ● Smear checks

   ● HIV prevention

   ● Masturbation

- Not getting pregnant
- Loving and caring
- Understanding
- Flirting
- Safer sex relationships – with other women if I choose

5 Still in the main group, ask women to think about the question, 'What has assertiveness to do with my sexual health?' Answers may include:

- Looking after myself
- Being able to say no and not feel guilty
- Pampering myself for once
- Asking for what I want
- Talking with my partner about what I want and need
- Putting my own needs first
- Being able to stand up to other people's prejudices

Discussion

End the session with a group discussion linking sexual health and women's ability to be assertive with future or past sessions. Explain how sessions on saying no, self-esteem and confidence may help women to become more assertive in their sexual lives.

Issues raised

- Facilitators should ensure that all group members understand the terms being used in the lists drawn up as part of this exercise (safer sex, for example, may be a new term for some women). You will also need to keep an eye on words like 'promiscuity'. (What does it mean? Someone who has more sex than me? Is it relative?)

- The final list the group draws up ('What has assertiveness to do with my sexual health?') may be quite similar to the first one. You might need to explore the fact that beginning to look at one aspect of our health has an effect on the rest of it. If we can be more assertive about sexual health it may have a follow-on effect. This can generate a lot of discussion, so allow time for it to come up if necessary.

61 Whose body is it anyway?

EXERCISE

Purpose
To enable women to explore and develop a common vocabulary for sexual parts of the body.

Suitable for
Looking at the language used for sex and sexuality, and encouraging young women or women with learning difficulties to explore the basics of sexuality. It's also fun!

Materials
Large sheets of flipchart paper, pens, photos of women representing different ages, races, abilities, shapes, sizes, and so on.

Method
1   Put a large sheet of paper on the floor. With one woman lying on it, get another to draw around her with a thick pen.

2   Pin the outline up and get women to take turns in drawing on it what they feel are sexual parts.

3   Finish this part of the exercise by looking at the photos of women's bodies. Is the picture the group has drawn similar to those seen in media advertisements? How diverse are women's bodies in terms of shape and size?

4   Next, get women to list all the words they can think of for each of the sexual parts. Once you have four or five for each, discuss the ones women like and dislike and why. Then agree which ones to use in the group.

Variation
If the group prefers not to draw round somebody, prepare an outline of a woman's body on a large sheet of paper beforehand. You could also prepare drawings of sexual body parts to stick on during the exercise (and have some blank pieces of paper in case women come up with others).

Discussion
Discuss why so many words used to describe women, their sexual parts and their sexualities are negative, and what we can do about them, if anything. What effect do they have on our confidence and self-esteem?

Issues raised

Facilitators need to be aware that some women may be embarrassed by drawing round each other, or drawing pictures of sexual body parts. You will need to work out, and perhaps discuss with the group, exactly what they feel comfortable with. Some women may be embarrassed or offended by the language or terms used by others in the group, especially if derogatory slang words are raised.

6J Messages

E X E R C I S E

Purpose

To encourage women to explore the messages and attitudes they have grown up with that have contributed to their views on sexuality.

Suitable for

Women of any age. This exercise often brings out some surprising information for women themselves, so do allow adequate time for reflection.

Materials

A copy of handout 6E for each woman, flipchart paper and lots of pens.

Method

1   Give each woman a copy of the handout. Ask them to think of sexual messages and attitudes to sex (both helpful and unhelpful ones) encountered at each stage of their life, then ask them to write or draw the messages on the handout in the appropriate age bracket. Point out that this exercise is not about being right or wrong about sex. Ensure that different cultural beliefs and values are treated with respect by the group. Women should be encouraged to draw their own conclusions from their own experiences.

2   Ask participants to pair up and discuss only those messages they want to clarify. How do these messages relate to their current ability to act assertively in sexual encounters?

Discussion

Give women plenty of time to share what has come up for them from this exercise.

Issues raised

This exercise can make women feel uncomfortable so it is important to check at the end how they are feeling, and perhaps to wind up with a positive message or a relaxation exercise to lighten things up.

6K Periods and the menopause

E X E R C I S E

Purpose

To enable participants to share their thoughts and feelings about starting and finishing their periods.

Suitable for

Women with learning difficulties, or, with modifications, young or older women. This is also a good exercise for a group of mixed age: the experiences of different women can be invaluable in opening up understanding of the processes of puberty and menopause.

Materials

A copy of handout 6F for each woman, pens.

Method

1   Discuss words women use to describe their periods and the images that they have of themselves when having or finishing their periods.

2   Give out the handout, and ask each participant to fill it in and then discuss with a partner the issues it raises for her.

Discussion

Develop a group discussion on the main points that have arisen. How do these relate to assertiveness? You could also explore attitudes to periods ('the curse', young women being told that problems with their periods will 'clear up' when they have a baby) and attitudes to the menopause. How are they viewed differently by men and by women? Draw on the group's experiences for this discussion.

Issues raised

The following points were made by one of the groups of women with learning difficulties taking part in the Project, and give some idea of what might come up in this part of the exercise.

● Most participants had been completely unprepared for the onset of their periods and the menopause. They had often felt scared and confused about both events. You should therefore emphasise the importance of gaining knowledge about our bodies, and give women the opportunity to ask questions and talk openly about what is often a taboo subject even with other women.

● Encouraging women to gain confidence to ask questions and obtain more information about their bodies inevitably means acknowledging that any change (for better or worse) also equals loss as well as gain – loss of childhood/ gain of fertility; loss of fertility/gain of freedom from fear of unwanted pregnancy or painful periods. Having acknowledged the difficult, painful or traumatic things associated with these changes, women can then be encouraged to celebrate their growth from child to woman and pre- to post-menopause.

6L Pleasurable experiences

E X E R C I S E

Purpose
To practise negotiation and promote discussion on what constitutes pleasurable experiences.

Suitable for
A group that knows each other well.

Materials
Some cards with one item from the list below written on each.

● Long hot bath

● Massaging hands

● Physical exercise

● Oral sex (giving or receiving)

● Listening to music

● Having a whole body massage

● Lying in the sun

● Foot massage

- Having shoulders and neck massaged
- Taking a sauna
- Relaxing in the shade
- Orgasm during sex
- Masturbation
- Eating chocolate
- Drinking champagne

Method

1 Ask each woman to choose a card without looking.

2 The whole group should then arrange themselves into a line in order of the level of pleasure that they all feel would be derived from each of the suggestions on the cards. Stress that they are not to apply any pressure and that they must negotiate with other women to find the right position.

3 The object of the exercise is to practise negotiation and promote discussion – not to get the positions absolutely right.

Discussion

1 End the exercise with a group discussion on what it was like to do the exercise. What issues did women come up with?

2 You could also ask women to express how they feel about the position they ended up in – feelings of envy, anger, rejection or competition may come up. This could lead into a discussion about assertiveness and not getting what you want.

Issues raised

When this exercise was used in the Project, participants who had chosen sexual activities arranged themselves in the order in which the activities would take place when a couple were making love – in the culturally conventional sense of the orgasm being the aim of sex. All other activities were placed in order according to whether they should take place before or after the 'event'.

This then led to a discussion on foreplay and negotiation: can foreplay be pleasurable in its own right? Is orgasm always the aim of sex?

6M Negotiating sex

EXERCISE

Purpose

To enable women to explore different kinds of relationships and then to focus on negotiating sexual relationships.

Suitable for

- Work with young women on sexual health and relationships.

- Women with teenagers who want to explore issues their children may be facing.

Materials

Pieces of paper, pens, and a small box or hat.

Method

1   Brainstorm 'relationships' by asking the group to come up with all the different combinations of relationships we have in our lives – male–female; female–female; male–male. Which kinds of people might these relationships involve (family, friends, colleagues, neighbours, pets, and so on)?

2   Ask each woman to write on a piece of paper what 'being in love' means to her. Put the pieces of paper in the hat/box and get everyone to pick one out and read it.

3   In pairs, ask women to discuss how we know we are in love with someone. Do we have to be 'in love' to have sex with someone? Explain that you are now going to move on to looking at negotiating sex with partners.

4   Now get women to begin to look at negotiating sex:

- What does virginity mean?

- How and when can it be lost?

- How do you know when and if it is right to lose it within a sexual relationship?

5   Get the group to feed back on what has been discussed. Now get women to brainstorm all the lines people use when asking for sex, and the possible responses. This can be fun and produces lots of good insights.

Discussion

Discuss any issues raised, for example:

- Do women negotiate sex or is it something that 'just happens'? What are the difficulties in negotiating sex?

- What prevents women from asking for sex?

- How do we choose to have sex with people (men or women)? How easy or difficult is it for us to be able to say no to the kinds of sex we don't want?

Issues raised

You could follow this session with one which looks at negotiating different forms of contraception, although this may not be appropriate for all groups (lesbians, for example).

6N Relationships

E X E R C I S E

Purpose

To develop discussion on sexual relationships.

Suitable for

Groups which have already covered some sexual health issues, or which already have a good level of trust. It's also a good exercise to use with young women – who may be at a stage in their lives when they see relationships as having only a 'sexual' focus.

Materials

Flipchart paper and pens.

Method

1 Brainstorm with the group all the types of relationships they can think of. Write these up on the flipchart. What do we mean by the word 'relationship'? How is a sexual relationship different from other kinds?

2 Split women into smaller groups and ask them to look at what makes a good sexual relationship and what makes a difficult sexual relationship. You could do this in two groups, each looking at one kind only. Ask the groups to think about 'good' and 'difficult' elements in relationships – none is completely one way or the other.

Discussion

Feed back in the main group. Discuss the following points:

- Can you recognise any of these elements in your close relationships?

- Is it possible to improve a difficult sexual relationship? How?

- How can we act assertively in difficult sexual relationships?

You could then use this exercise as a trigger for discussions on how to be assertive in relationships.

Issues raised

An exercise of this nature could make women feel very emotional. If someone feels that all her relationships are difficult and can see no way of changing them, she may need counselling or group support to explore the issue further. Facilitators should concentrate on keeping group discussions balanced, reaffirming ground rules and, where necessary, referring women to local agencies.

60 Difficulties in expressing our sexual needs

E X E R C I S E

Purpose

To enable participants to explore their feelings and thoughts about their sexual needs.

Suitable for

Groups who have built up a good level of trust and are familiar with issues around sexual health and assertiveness.

Materials

A copy of handout 6G for each woman. Flipchart and pens.

Method

1 Give out copies of the handout. Ask women to pair up and identify things that would make them feel comfortable or uncomfortable. Explain that the handout is geared, to some extent, to women in heterosexual relationships (point 13, for example) but that most of it is applicable to any sexual relationship.

2 Ask the group to brainstorm their fears or concerns about expressing sexual needs. The group might come up with some of the following answers:

- Risk of being accused of being promiscuous, a 'slut' or a 'prick-teaser'

- Media influences – stereotypes of women who do express their sexual needs

- Women are not expected to initiate sexual activity or have sexual needs

- Upbringing

- Mistrust

- Questions will be asked if I want to try something new or negotiate different contraception ('where did she learn this?')

- Lack of confidence to ask

- Lack of awareness

- Uncertainty about whose needs are being met

Discussion

Discuss with the group some of the issues raised. For example:

- How can inability to express our needs in these areas affect our health and lives?

- How can women assert themselves in expressing their sexual needs?

Issues raised

You may want to discuss with the group how being assertive about sexual needs can raise new challenges and problems in relationships. Are women willing, able or ready to take these risks? What would they do if they were rejected, judged or put down as a result of the new steps they might take?

(Many thanks to Rose Brown, HIV Prevention Officer at North Derbyshire Health Authority, for additional information on the assertiveness ladder.)

6P Safer sex

EXERCISE

Purpose

To enable women to find out what safer sex means to them.

Suitable for

- Encouraging women to share and develop their perceptions of the term 'safer sex'.

- An introduction to exercises on negotiating sex, such as exercise 6M. Exercises like this should be used only after ground rules around trust and confidentiality have been established.

Materials

Flipchart paper and pens. You may also want to read in advance, or share with the group, leaflets and resources relevant to safer sex.

Method

1 Begin with a discussion on what women in the group already know about the term 'safer sex'.

2 Next, divide the group into two and ask one group to brainstorm, 'Sex is . . .' and the other to brainstorm, 'Safer sex is . . .'.

3 Now ask the whole group to explore what prevents them having safer sex. Be mindful that some women in the group may feel safer sex is irrelevant to them – they may be celibate, for example. Chart the responses on flipchart paper.

4 Once you have made your lists, get the group to try and come up with a definition that encompasses what they feel safer sex is for them.

Discussion

Finish with a discussion on what it was like to do an exercise like this. This kind of exercise often includes discussion on equality in relationships or negotiating sex that does not involve a penis entering the vagina (non-penetrative sex) so do allow adequate time to talk through the issues.

Issues raised

● This exercise often throws up interesting distinctions: sex is sometimes seen as dangerous, exciting or dirty; safer sex is about methods – condoms, massage, and so on. It's easy to assume that people know what safer sex means. It is often thought of as relevant only to HIV, rather than about talking with your partner, for example, about how to protect each other from all sexually transmitted diseases or, if relevant, unplanned pregnancy. Women may feel nervous of broaching the subject, but most people feel relieved when their partner (male or female) shows concern and starts off the conversation.

● Some women may consider safer sex irrelevant to them – in reality it may not be. The discussion could be directed towards STDs and behaviour that risks infection and whether or not anyone who is sexually active can afford to ignore safer sex.

6Q Negotiating condom use

EXERCISE

Purpose

To enable women to gain experience of dealing with their partners' refusal to use condoms.

Suitable for

Young women, or women who are concerned about beginning new relationships because of the risk of HIV/AIDS, STDs, unplanned pregnancy, and so on. Use it after you have looked at the difference between assertive, aggressive and passive behaviour (exercise 1F). This exercise needs to come at a stage when trust has been established. Participants need to feel safe about exploring this issue personally. Be sensitive and aware of the group's needs – you might want to give 'dental dam'/'oral shield' as an alternative to condom.

Materials

None.

Method

1 Remind women of the differences between asssertive, aggressive and passive behaviour which the group has already looked at.

2 Ask women to divide into pairs. Tell them that you are going to give them some examples of things people say when discussing condom use; and that the purpose of this exercise is not to get the lines right, but to practise getting our needs met in sexual situations.

3 • Ask Woman A to say to Woman B: 'I want you to use a condom.'

• Woman B should then say: 'You want me to use a condom?'

• Woman A should then say: 'Yes' – assertively; aggressively (include manipulatively); passively.

• Woman B should then say either: 'But I don't like using condoms'; or 'Don't you trust me?'

• Woman A should then reply, assertively: 'But I want to use a condom for my health and yours'; or 'Yes, but I don't want to have sex without a condom.'

4 Now, ask women to swap around so that Woman B is asking Woman A to use a condom.

5 If appropriate, you could work on negotiating other safer sex alternatives – 'I don't want to have sex with you inside me', for example.

Discussion

1 Discuss ways in which women could respond to partners' unwillingness or refusal to practise safer sex and/or how they might deal with partners refusing their request to use a condom. Do we start from an equal footing in relationships? How does this affect our ability to communicate what we want?

2 What are our expectations of sexual relationships? Would women who are in violent or oppressive relationships be able to use anything from this exercise?

3 End by pointing out that being able to negotiate is part of a process of change. It can sometimes have unexpected results – perhaps rejection. You need to reassure women that these discussions only offer suggestions for dealing with issues in their lives; it is up to them to decide whether they feel able to apply them.

Issues raised

Within the Project this exercise proved to be constructive and lots of fun. It can get complicated if participants are not clear about the difference between aggressive, passive and assertive responses so ensure that the group has covered this. It may also be good to redefine these behaviours in the context of the exercise.

The exercise can also lead to discussions about how long women should continue using condoms with a 'new' partner – when is a partner not 'new'? It might help to suggest materials giving information on safer sex and where to go for advice, to help women make informed choices.

6R Looking at contraception

E X E R C I S E

Purpose

To enable women to negotiate different kinds of contraception using the assertiveness skills they have already gained.

Suitable for

Heterosexual groups who have already looked at negotiating relationships, and have built up a good level of trust.

Materials

Flipchart paper, pens.

Method

1 Get women to brainstorm different forms of contraception, writing each one on a different piece of paper. What are the advantages and disadvantages of each method?

2 Divide the group into pairs and give each pair one or two forms of contraception to look at. How would women discuss using these forms of contraception with their partners?

Discussion

Get the small groups to feed back their thoughts. Are women already using assertiveness to get their contraceptive needs met? How might being assertive help those who aren't? What are the issues when discussing different forms of contraception in a relationship? Does this depend on the kind of relationship it is?

Issues raised

Groups might want to look at the boundaries between safer sex and contraception. Be sensitive to different cultural or religious conditions – taboos around contraception, family size, women's ability to take control of their own fertility. Facilitators should ensure they are appropriately informed about contraceptive choices and are ready to challenge myths and stereotypes.

6S Ending relationships

E X E R C I S E

Purpose

To enable women to explore the difficulties involved in ending relationships.

Suitable for

Young women. Within the Project, this exercise was carried out with a group of 15–16-year-old women, about half of whom were in relationships they did not want to be in. Think carefully about whether to use this exercise with women who may find the results of ending relationships very traumatic. For these women, the costs and benefits of such a step must be considered.

Materials

Flipchart paper, pens.

Method

1 Begin with a discussion on how much choice we have when we enter a relationship. What influences us in our choice of partners? If we are not happy, what choices do we have to bring about change?

2 Ask the group to list the reasons for not ending relationships. Write these up on the flipchart.

3 Ask the group to think about each of these reasons. How could they argue against them? How might they end relationships assertively?

Discussion

Encourage participants to practise role-playing ending relationships in ways that would feel assertive to them. Close by discussing how it felt to practise different ways of ending relationships and how practical they would be in reality. Discuss their advantages and disadvantages. Do they have anything in common?

Issues raised

It is important to be aware of the implications that looking at ending relationships might have. You need to make sure that the group recognises different types of relationship – arranged marriages, lesbian relationships, cross-cultural partnerships, and so on. The group may want to discuss issues relating to parental/family pressure, or breaking religious codes, all of which have considerable effects on women's self-image, status in their peer group, and their degree of acceptance in the community.

6T Group massage

EXERCISE

Purpose

To enable women to experience giving and receiving physical contact.

Suitable for

Groups that have been meeting for some time and have developed trust. This exercise may not be appropriate for wheelchair users or for anyone who has difficulty sitting on the floor, unless they feel comfortable enough with the group to be supported during the exercise.

Materials

None.

Method

1   Get the group to sit in a circle on the floor, all facing the same way, so that each woman has her back to the woman behind.

2   Each woman should then gently massage the back and shoulders of the woman in front.

Discussion

After a few moments get the group to relax for a short while. Ask them how the exercise felt. Lead on to a discussion about asking for what we want in terms of physical contact. Do we know what we want, or do we just accept or reject what we get?

Issues raised

Care needs to be taken when using exercises involving touch. Women may, for a variety of reasons, feel unable or unwilling to participate in exercises of this nature. Do ask women about this, beforehand, and respect their wishes if they don't want to be involved.

6A What does being healthy mean to me?

Tick any of the following statements that are important aspects of health for you.

- Enjoying being with my family and friends

- Living to a ripe old age

- Feeling cheerful and optimistic most of the time

- Being able to make a decision without dithering

- Hardly ever taking tablets or medicines

- Being the ideal weight for my height

- Taking part in lots of sport

- Feeling at peace with myself

- Never smoking

- Having clear skin, bright eyes, shiny hair

- Never suffering from anything more serious than a mild cold or stomach upset

- Not getting things confused or out of proportion – assessing situations realistically

Handout 6A

© Health Education Authority, 1994: photocopiable

- Being able to adapt easily to changes in my life – moving house, changing jobs, partners, and so on

- Feeling glad to be alive when I wake up in the morning

- Drinking only moderate amounts of alcohol, or none at all

- Enjoying my work without much stress or strain

- Having a healthy body

- Getting on well with other people most of the time

- Eating the 'right' foods

- Enjoying some form of relaxation or recreation

- Hardly ever going to the doctor

6B What affects my health?

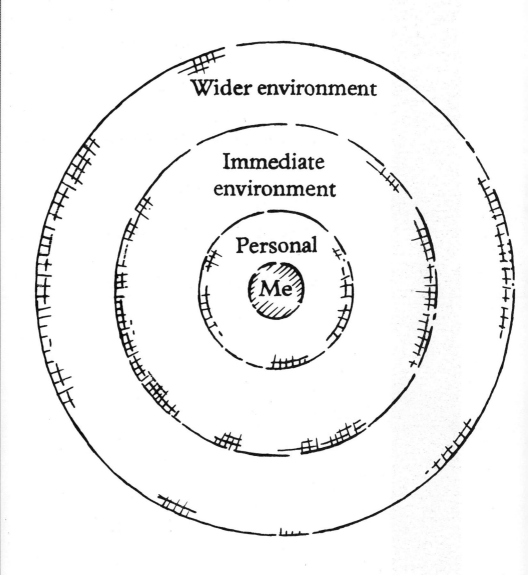

Wider environment

Immediate environment

Personal

Me

6C Things in my life . . .

. . . that help me to be healthy	. . . that stop me from being healthy

6D Asking for what I want

- At the chemist's

- At the doctor's for advice on:
    - giving up smoking
    - cutting down on drinking
    - choosing what to eat

- Getting housing

- Dealing with legal professionals

- Asking a partner to use a condom or an oral shield

- Asking for sex more or less often with a partner

- Asking for different sex which might be more exciting or pleasurable

- Asking for a massage

- Asking for a hug

- Any others?

6E Messages

Age	Sexual messages and attitudes to sex
0–5 years	
6–10 years	
11–15 years	
16–20 years	
21–30 years	
31–40 years	
41–50 years	
51+ years	

6F Periods

What happens to me when I have a period?

Periods are . . .

The first time I found out about periods was . . .

The first time I had my period I felt . . .

When/if my periods stopped, I felt/would feel . . .

6G Assertiveness ladder

17 Suggesting that we use a vibrator or sex toy.

16 Suggesting that I show my partner, by masturbating, how I can be turned on more easily.

15 Saying I want to make love without intercourse.

14 Telling my partner that I have often pretended to have an orgasm.

13 Asking my partner to delay penetration.

12 Telling my partner that I did not have an orgasm and that I do not want one just now.

11 Asking my partner to talk when making love.

10 Telling my partner that something he or she does is uncomfortable.

9 Saying I don't want to make love.

8 Suggesting a change in the way we make love.

7 Saying that I don't like something my partner is doing.

6 Getting my partner to realise how switched off I am when we have been disturbed.

5 Describing the effects of something we are doing together.

4 Saying what I would like my partner to do.

3 Describing my sexual feelings.

2 Explaining to my partner changes in desire at different times of the month.

1 Saying I enjoy something my partner is doing.

Adapted from *Woman's experience of sex* (Penguin)

7 Rights and responsibilities

Exploring women's rights and responsibilities in relation to health proved to be particularly useful to many of the groups who took part in the Project. Women often find it easier to take control when they see their rights written down, as if having them in print legitimises them. Several women said that they had put copies up on the fridge or wall as a constant reminder to themselves (and their families) that they are individuals too.

These exercises offer women great opportunities to make changes and become more healthy in their lives, but it is important to stress that this is not a substitute for changes in others and in society itself. Sometimes it is appropriate for women to choose (assertively) not to assert themselves – they alone can judge these kinds of situations.

You should try to acknowledge the context of different women's lives. It may be possible to identify rights and responsibilities, but it may not be so easy to assert them. It is also important to look at how women feel about other people in their lives having the same rights.

One of the best ways of working in this area is to encourage women to develop their own health rights, which are realistic and relevant to their lives and cultures. The following materials should be used as ideas on which to base the development of a group's own health rights.

7A What are my rights?

EXERCISE

Purpose
To encourage women to develop their own ideas of what their rights are.

Suitable for
Groups that have already established trust and confidence in each other. Women need to feel safe to express themselves when exploring what can often be a difficult subject.

Materials
Flipchart paper and pens. A copy of the rights lists of your choice (either handout 7A or 7B) for each woman, and a single copy of the success story (handout 7C).

123

Method

1 Working together, brainstorm and write up on flipchart paper what women feel that every woman has the right to – the right to make mistakes, the right to her own opinion, and so on. Explain that at this stage you want the group to think realistically about this but not to start discussing any limitations raised by the examples.

2 Divide into small groups and give out one of the rights handouts. Ask the groups to:

- compare this list with the one drawn up by the large group;

- note similarities and differences;

- discuss how easy or difficult it would be for women to feel these rights applied to them, and why;

- discuss what the implications might be of asserting these rights – having the right to say yes or no in a sexual relationship, for example;

- discuss what happens if we are denied these rights.

Discussion

Bring the groups back together and ask women to summarise their thoughts. To end the session, either read out the success story or ask someone in the group to tell one of her own.

Issues raised

Issues that may emerge could include young people's right to stand up for themselves and challenge other people's behaviour, or women's right to dress as they want to. It is important to discuss the implications that awareness of these issues may have on women's lives and behaviour. (Other people – family members, for example – may find their assertiveness threatening and try to put them down.)

7B Rights and choices

EXERCISE

Purpose

- To enable women to identify the choices they have and the rights they need to assert to make those choices.

- To enable women to explore how they feel about according these rights to others.

Suitable for

Groups where there is a low level of literacy. Exercises where you can lay the material out on the floor or a table for women to choose are nearly always popular, and this one also gives women something tangible to take away with them. This exercise also builds on earlier exercises on self-esteem.

Materials
- Cut out balloon shapes and write down rights on them, one on each shape (use rights you have developed with the group, or one of the lists of rights (handout 7A or 7B)).
- Copies of the rights lists (handouts 7A and 7B) to give out at the end of the session.

Method
1 Put the completed rights balloons on the floor or table and ask each woman to pick up the one(s) that are particularly important to her.

2 Get women to pair up and talk about the importance of these particular rights.

Discussion
1 Discuss in the main group how, if we accept these rights for ourselves, we must also acknowledge that others have them too.

2 You could also look at the right to waive our rights if appropriate, and the importance of negotiating and thinking through the consequences of decisions.

3 Where does assertiveness fit into possessing rights? How would women negotiate maintaining their own rights (and recognising those of others) without being aggressive? Make sure women have copies of the rights lists to take home.

You could end the exercise by asking women to write or dictate a letter to themselves which you, the facilitator will post in three months' time. These should begin, 'Dear . . . By the time I receive this letter I will have [list 5 things].' The letter should end, 'I am going to treat myself to . . .'. Get women to think of things which will enable them to assert the rights they have already identified.

Issues raised
- Women are often surprised at the rights they choose to pick out during this exercise. (For example, a nurse picked

out 'I have the right to be ill' because she saw herself as always being a carer whatever her own state of health.)

- If this exercise is used with health service workers or social work staff they may be concerned about abusing their position of authority. They may, for instance, feel that they have the right to say no to their clients – but not too often. Discussing women's right to waive their rights if they feel uncomfortable would be particularly relevant in this type of group.

7C Saying no

EXERCISE

Purpose

To encourage awareness of the range of behaviour employed when making requests or saying no, and the detrimental effects on our health.

Suitable for

Highlighting the ease with which people switch from one behaviour pattern to another, particularly when they are trying to persuade somebody to do something. This exercise can be a lot of fun and could be quite active. If there are wheelchair users in the group, ensure that they are able to manoeuvre around the room, or that other women can change around to work with them with the minimum of fuss.

Materials

Flipchart paper and pens; a copy of handout 7D for each woman. Enough physical space to arrange two circles of chairs, one facing out and one in.

Method

1 Ask the group to give examples (related to their health) of people or situations they find it difficult to say 'no' to. It may be a good idea if you give an example of your own here as a starting point (saying no to chocolate, medical treatment, and so on).

2 Write their examples up on flipchart paper under the heading, 'I find it hard to say no to . . .'. They might include:

- Chocolate when depressed or alone

- Charity collectors at Christmas

- Family

- Alcohol when pregnant

- Salespeople
- Treatment when I am ill
- Friends
- Doctor

As you chart up each of the examples ask how being unable to say no to these specifically affects women's health.

3 Once you have several examples ask women to arrange their chairs into a carousel (with half the group placing their chairs in a circle facing out and the other half facing in). Now ask women on the inside circle to pick a topic from the list you have just drawn up. Their job is to persuade the women on the outside to say yes; but the women on the outside must keep refusing.

4 Do this once (allowing about three minutes) then move women in one of the circles two spaces to the left. Ask women to sit down facing their new partner. This time women on the outside pick a topic from the list and those on the inside say no. Ask women to make a note of how it feels to ask and be refused, and to keep saying no.

5 Do steps 3 and 4 once or twice more, changing back and forth, and asking women to choose a topic that relates specifically to them.

6 Next divide the women into two groups (the inner circle could be one and the outer circle another). Give each group a sheet of paper and ask them to write down:

- all the methods of persuasion they used in this exercise or that were used on them;
- all the ways they and others used to say no;
- the possible effects on their health of not saying no.

Variation
Instead of drawing up a list, use cards with examples already written on them and give out different ones to the 'persuaders' in each round of the activity.

Discussion
Discuss as a group what comes up as a result of these lists. What is the best way to say no? Give women the handout to consolidate the exercise.

7D Saying no assertively

E X E R C I S E

Purpose

To give women the opportunity of experiencing saying no aggressively, passively and assertively, and to look at how this can affect their health.

Suitable for

This is a quick exercise which could be used on its own or as a possible follow-up to reinforce learning about the differences between aggressive, passive and assertive behaviour (see handout 1B). Because this exercise requires movement, you will need to be sensitive to women who may have physical difficulties standing for any length of time. The exercise can be done sitting or standing, so discuss with the group how they wish to do it beforehand.

Materials

None.

Method

1   Ask women to find a space in the room where they feel at ease. Get them to relax and to stand or sit with their feet slightly apart. Ask them to breathe deeply in through the nose and out through the mouth and to imagine a thread running from the top of their head to the base of their spine – their backs should be as straight and flexible as possible. Ask them to continue to breathe deeply and to make eye contact with others, avoiding smiling.

2   Get the women to choose someone to work with. They should then stand or sit opposite their partners, forming two rows. Determining their own distances, maintaining their composure and avoiding physical contact, one partner says yes whilst the other says no. Each time, women should try a different way of speaking – passively or aggressively. How does each of these words feel?

3   Women then try to say yes or no assertively, and convince each other that they mean yes or no. Ask women to note the tone of voice and body language used.

Discussion

1   Focus a group discussion on how it felt to say yes and no passively, aggressively and assertively. You could then look at the health implications of speaking in a particular way. Saying no aggressively might feel OK in the short term

but could lead to unhealthy relationships and feeling bad in the long term.

2 Discuss what happens when saying no or making a request assertively does not make any difference – if someone ignores the request, or, for example, overrides their sexual wishes.

Issues raised

Women may at first feel silly saying yes and no. You need to acknowledge this and explain again the purpose of doing exercises like this, which help women to gain a deeper understanding of their own and others' behaviour.

7E Broken record technique

E X E R C I S E

'Broken record' is the name given to an assertiveness technique that is particularly useful when you know what you want. It involves deciding what it is you want to say, choosing a clear and direct statement that conveys what you want to communicate to the other person, and then sticking to it even in the face of argument.

Purpose

To demonstrate and practise the broken record assertiveness technique in order to give women a skill for use in situations generally, and in relation to their health in particular.

Suitable for

Use after sessions on body language and self-esteem so that women can translate what they have learned from those sessions into a particular technique.

Materials

Flipchart or board, pens.

Method

1 Write on the flipchart or board the following example of an exchange between a patient and a consultant (BR = broken record).

BR: I want more information about this treatment.

Answer: I have given you as much as I think is necessary.

BR: I would like more information about this treatment.

Answer: Well, women don't usually want to know any more.

BR: *I want more information about this treatment.*

2 Point out the slight variation each time, either in words or in emphasis. Look at potential trouble spots where the woman making the request could get caught up in an argument or go off the track. She could, for instance, get caught by saying, 'I don't want to be a nuisance.' This leaves the door wide open for the consultant to say something like, 'Oh no, not at all. Now, where were we?' which would make it difficult to start again with a request for more information.

3 Ask women to think of a situation affecting their health where they could use the broken record technique – with a GP or consultant, with a friend or family member, at school, at home, at work, and so on.

4 Divide the group into threes. Each woman should then take a turn at exploring with the others how she could use the broken record technique in her situation. Ask women, still in their threes, to practise their interchanges, with two 'coaching' the other one on body language, tone of voice, and facial expression, as well as the actual words used.

Discussion

Close by bringing everyone back to the main group. Ask each woman to say a little about the situation she has been practising and to state the sentence(s) she would use if the situation were to arise again.

Issues raised

- In the Project, one group of young women found this technique very useful and was able to adapt it to many different situations – friends making excessive demands, for example.

- For many young women, having the courage and the confidence to persist with a response to an unreasonable request can be very difficult. Peer pressure and social situations involving drink and/or drugs can undermine their confidence to resist unwanted demands. This technique provides a useful, yet simple, tool to help them deal with such situations.

- This exercise focused many of the more 'theoretical'

discussions the group had had earlier in the course (about
talking to themselves, self-confidence, non-verbal
communication, and so on). Women were able to
appreciate the real meaning and benefits of behaving
assertively. Many expressed a feeling of greater confidence
in trying to be assertive as a result of learning this
technique.

7A Rights list 1

- I have the right to be treated with respect as an intelligent, capable and equal human being.

- I have the right to express my feelings.

- I have the right to express my opinions and values.

- I have the right to say no or yes for myself.

- I have the right to make mistakes.

- I have the right to change my mind.

- I have the right to say 'I don't understand', and to ask for more information.

- I have the right to ask for what I want.

- I have the right to decline responsibility for other people's problems.

- I have the right to deal with others without being dependent on them for approval.

- I have the right to state my own needs and set my own priorities as a person, independent of any roles that I may assume in my life.

7B Rights list 2

- The right to say no
- The right to relax
- The right to my own time and space
- The right to be independent
- The right to be respected as a person
- The right to a social life
- The right to choose
- The right not to be judged
- The right to be listened to and heard
- The right to make mistakes
- The right to my own opinion
- The right to change my mind
- The right to the best health care available
- The right to make decisions about my life
- The right to freedom of movement – to go where I want
- The right to have my views respected
- The right to be unwell and to get well
- The right to grieve
- The right to my feelings
- The right to decide what to do with my own body, property and time
- The right not to take responsibility for other people's problems

7C Success story

A young woman with two small children was able to make use of her rights to change a dental appointment. She needed a return visit and an appointment was offered to her at lunchtime. This would have meant that she would have to pick up her eldest child from playschool, go home, be at home for 10–15 minutes then leave for the dental appointment.

In-between she would have to take off and put on the baby's padded suit, upset her eldest by having just got in and then going out, and so on. However, she decided to use the rights discussed in the session to ask for a different appointment at a more convenient time.

She was surprised and delighted to achieve a positive result – an appointment which fitted in with playschool and childcare arrangements. She said that she would never have considered asking for the appointment to be changed if rights had not been covered in the session. Instead she would have struggled to fit everything in and deal with the stress around it.

7D Gut reaction

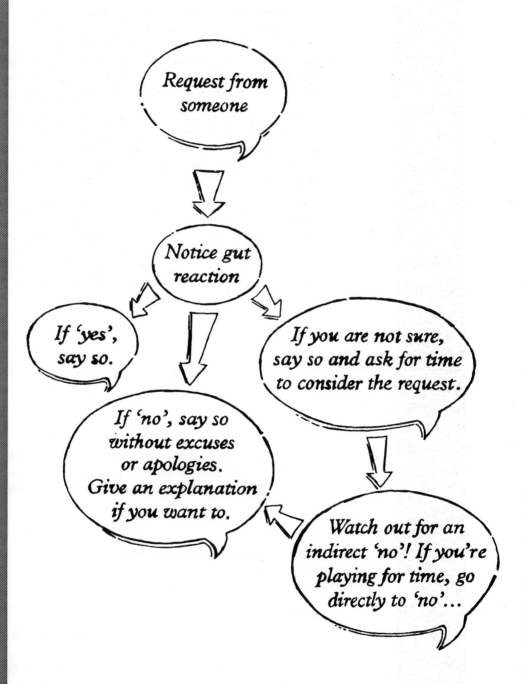

8 Anger

Anger is an emotion that many women are reluctant to confront. It occupies a lot of unhealthy space in our lives, both on an internal, personal level and more generally. Anger is not just about shouting or being aggressive – it can also leave us feeling defeated, frustrated, powerless and passive.

However, anger can also be harnessed positively, and can often provide a motivation for action. This is important on a personal level and is particularly so for groups and individuals campaigning against inequality and injustice.

The illustration opposite outlines a number of issues relating to anger and health, and was developed by a group of women in Bradford on a course run by a woman from the Project.

8A Anger, health and assertiveness

EXERCISE

Purpose
To raise awareness of the links between anger and health and how assertiveness can alleviate the effects of anger.

Suitable for
Use with groups who have already spent some time with each other and have built up enough trust to enable them to explore these issues. Allow plenty of time for this exercise.

Materials
Flipchart paper and pens, copies of handouts 8A, 8B and 8C for each woman.

Method
1 Explain to women that becoming more assertive can alleviate the stress associated with anger by helping us to see that we have choices about how we respond to situations. The starting point for this exercise is to identify the physical and mental effects of being angry or of having anger directed at you.

2 Ask the group to say anything that comes into their heads

Anger

What makes us angry?

What can anger do to our health?

How does anger make us feel?

How do we deal with anger?
• In a healing way?
• In a destructive way?

How can we deal with our anger more effectively?
• Expressing our feelings?
• Saying no?
• Challenging criticisms and put-downs?
• Stopping the flow of anger

when you say the word 'anger', and write it up on flipchart paper. Examples might include:

- temper
- loss of control
- banging and stomping
- gritting teeth
- bad power
- nastiness
- frustration
- rage
- sighing
- sulking
- unreasonableness
- sarcasm

3 Next, ask the group what they think the health issues connected to anger are, and list what they come up with. Examples might include:

- stomach-turning
- can't eat
- change of facial colour
- high blood pressure
- sours relationships if kept inside/can ruin relationships if expressed
- violence

4 Discuss with the group what has come up as a result of these lists. Get women to pair up to start looking at how they deal with their own and other people's anger.

5 Give out handout 8A. Ask women to go through the list and explain to their partner which examples apply to them and in which situations they tend to happen.

6 Give out handout 8B. Ask women to spend a little time on their own filling out the sheet and then discuss their responses with their partner.

7 Give out handout 8C and ask participants to choose a situation where they have felt angry and to apply these guidelines to it. Get them to discuss with their partner what would be different if they were able to follow these

guidelines and what might stop them doing this in the future.

Variation 1

Prepare the charts on anger and the relevant health issues before the session, and ask women what they feel about them. Ask them to add things to the charts from their own experiences of feeling angry. Continue from step 4.

Variation 2

1   You could end the session at step 7 or, if you have enough time, you could add some work on body language and voice tone which would help to consolidate and extend learning for women.

2   Explain that when communicating anger (or anything else), it is very important to be aware of the part 'body language' plays: research has shown that when we communicate only 7 per cent of what is communicated comes from the words we choose; 33 per cent from the tone of voice; and a massive 60 per cent from our body language.

3   With this in mind ask women to get together with a partner and practise saying, 'I am really angry with you':

   •   in a loud voice

   •   in a whisper

   •   through gritted teeth

   •   with a smile

   •   firmly

   •   gently

4   End with a group discussion on how this felt and the best ways of expressing anger without giving mixed messages.

8B Exploring anger

EXERCISE

Purpose

To encourage women to look at expressing their feelings linked to anger.

Suitable for

Groups able to have constructive and honest discussions. If you have a big group, divide women into smaller groups for some of the questions and then have them feed back to the main group.

Materials
None.

Method

1 Begin by getting the group to discuss the statement: 'I have the right to express my feelings when I am angry.' Many women find it difficult to express their feelings because they are often seen as neurotic, emotional or aggressive. (For example, black women are often perceived as aggressive when they express how they feel about any grievances they may have.)

2 Looking at anger as a specific emotion or feeling, ask the group:

- What are your thoughts about anger?

- Which things make you angry?

- How do you deal with anger (your own and other people's)?

3 Then ask the group:

- What makes each of us respond differently to similar situations? (For example, when being shouted at, one woman may respond by crying, another by shouting back.)

- What thoughts and feelings come into play when we are angry?

- What happens to our health when anger is left unexpressed or expressed indirectly?

- How could anger be expressed positively?

Discussion

Ask the group to consider ways of handling anger more effectively using handout 8C. End the session with a relaxation exercise or a poem with a positive message so that women can let go of any negative feelings to do with anger before moving on.

Issues raised

The last part of this exercise may raise the issue that anger can be debilitating and exhausting (whether expressed or suppressed). If it is not resolved, it can cause headaches, tension, stomach upsets, arguments, and irritability.

8A When I am angry I'm...

(Tick those that apply to you.)

... uncomfortable

... worried

... calm

... afraid

... in control

... out of control

... clear-minded

... confused

... reasonable

... unreasonable

... outspoken

... loud

... quiet

... silent

... depressed

... relaxed

... tense

... aggressive

... any others?

8B Different kinds of anger

1 What feelings does anger stem from? (Hatred, resentment, jealousy, injustice, inequality?)

2 What happens to anger once it is felt? What do people do with their anger? (Suppress it? React violently?)

3 What else could people do with their anger? (Motivate themselves? Express it, so that it doesn't turn inwards on themselves, or outwards on more vulnerable people?)

4 Do you think anger can be constructive? Can you think of examples where you or others have used anger constructively?

5 When was the last time you felt angry? What happened? How did you feel? What did you do?

8C Assertiveness guidelines

1   Decide what you feel.

2   Decide what you want and what you want to say.

3   Say it clearly, directly and specifically ('I am angry with you for . . . , I feel . . . as a result, and I would like . . .). What you are doing here is blaming the behaviour, not the person, saying how you feel, and outlining what you would like to happen.

4   Don't lose track of what you are saying.

5   Give yourself time – you don't have to respond straight away.

9 Dealing with criticism

Many of us live with the effects of criticisms that have been made of us in the past. Perhaps we were called lazy as a child and now always think of ourselves in that way. Sometimes people exaggerate the original criticism and develop a distorted view of themselves. For example, a woman in her fifties in a group looking at criticism said, 'I am uneducated.' This criticism was then simply repeated to her: 'So, you are uneducated.' 'Well, it's not that, it's that I cannot spell.'

Not being able to spell is very different from being uneducated, and in fact there were only certain words that she could not spell. We often exaggerate criticism and generalise it until it alters the way we see our whole personality.

Criticism can be very stressful both to give and to receive. Feeling anxious about criticising someone can give us sleepless nights. Similarly, receiving criticism from others (constructive or otherwise) can be stressful, and negative or 'invalid' criticism can leave us feeling hurt, angry, rejected or confused – all of which have implications for our health.

Learning to deal with criticism, therefore, is an important step towards feeling good about ourselves and others. So how can women deal with criticism more effectively? The exercises in this section should help you to move through this area.

9A Living with self-criticism

E X E R C I S E

Purpose
To enable women to look at criticism of them in the past, and how to deal with it.

Suitable for
Early on in a course or group as an introduction to self-confidence and self-esteem.

Materials
A copy of handout 9A for each woman, pens.

Method
1   Divide the group into pairs, and give each woman a copy of

the handout. Ask women to spend time thinking about answers to the questions; then write them down and discuss them with their partners.

2   Get the pairs to feed back to the main group.

Discussion

Initiate a group discussion on how past criticism can affect the way we see ourselves. Why do we keep remembering these criticisms?

End by explaining that criticism made of us in the past is rarely valid now (it may not have been then either!) and that learning to let go of these negative messages is important.

Issues raised

Often women find that a lot of the criticism they live with has long ceased to have any real relevance to them – they have just never challenged these labels.

9B Facing criticism

E X E R C I S E

Purpose

To increase awareness about our reactions to being criticised.

Suitable for

A follow-on from the previous exercise. This one looks specifically at dealing with criticism from others.

Materials

A copy of the handout 9B for each woman, pens.

Method

Split the group into pairs or fours. Ask each group to go through the handout, identifying what their reactions are to criticism.

Discussion

Bring the group back together to discuss the following issues.

● How do we react to others' criticisms of us? Do we re-act (act again) those criticisms? Do we re-enact responses to previous criticisms?

● What feelings does criticism raise?

- Can we change our behaviour? How? Would it be useful to role-play some of these critical situations? (Leave enough time for this.)

- How can we resolve to behave differently in future?

Issues raised

People generally want to avoid conflict, and therefore avoid responding honestly and effectively to criticism. They may feel embarrassed, want to cry, or shout. Therefore it's important to look at how women can acknowledge and then deal with these feelings and explore ways of dealing with the *criticism* rather than the *feelings* it provokes.

9C Dealing with criticism

E X E R C I S E

Purpose

To enable women to begin to distinguish between valid and invalid criticism.

Suitable for

A group that feels safe and supportive, and able to be honest with themselves and others.

Materials

A copy of handout 9C for each woman, pens.

Method

1 Ask women to fill in the handout individually. Allow five minutes.

2 Ask women to pair up and swap handouts. In turn, each woman should read out, with conviction, her partner's first 'untrue criticism'. The partner should then listen to the criticism and react by saying something like, 'I don't think I am/do . . .'. Women should note how they feel about this exchange.

3 Once each partner has reacted to her first 'definitely untrue criticisms', women should carry on down the list – reacting to 'sometimes true criticisms' by saying something like, 'Yes, I am sometimes'; and to 'true criticisms' by something like, 'Yes, you're right' or 'That's perfectly true.' Each time, women should note how they feel.

Discussion

Bring the group back together and discuss some of the
following issues.

1 What does it feel like (a) to be the person giving the
   criticism? (b) to be receiving it and responding?

2 What might the long-term effects be on your health and
   self-esteem if you are always being criticised unfairly?

End by asking women to 'dump' their invalid criticisms in an
imaginary well in the middle of the room or to shake them off
physically as a symbolic way of 'getting rid' of them.

Issues raised

Women are often unsure about how to overcome their
'natural' or 'learned' reactions to criticism (such as
automatically assuming the criticism must be valid). Encourage
them to look beyond these reactions and to practise responding
differently, even if it feels alien and uncomfortable. Be aware
that the indirect effects of criticism on women's health may
also come up in discussion, such as being victims of physical
violence or emotional blackmail.

9A What we say to ourselves

1   What three things don't you like about yourself?

2   What do you say to yourself/do about these things?

3   Where did this criticism come from? Can you remember who said it to you, and why?

4   Is it valid? Is it still true today?

5   How does it make you feel? What effect does it have on your physical and emotional health?

9B Reacting to criticism

Someone criticises you or what you're doing.
How do you feel?

How do you react?

What do you say?

What do you do?

Does your body language change? How?

Does it make a difference if the criticism is valid or invalid?

9C Valid and invalid

Three criticisms which people make of me which are definitely not true:

1

2

3

Three criticisms which people make of me which might be true sometimes:

1

2

3

Three criticisms which people make of me which are true:

1

2

3

Exercise section II
For black women's groups

10 Taking part

For black women, it can be difficult to come along to meetings, events and groups. They may require specific encouragement and support to attend. There will probably be practical barriers: women may need to negotiate time with employers or families, for example. There may also be more 'hidden' difficulties: issues about working in groups with other black women, perhaps.

Although groups can be a good opportunity for black women to learn how to improve their own health and well-being, you will need to address attendance and participation concerns first. The following exercise will enable you to do this.

10A Addressing participation concerns

EXERCISE

Purpose
To begin to explore and find ways of addressing difficulties black women experience in taking part in groups.

Suitable for
Beginning a group.

Materials
A copy of handout 10A for each woman, pens, flipchart paper.

Method
1   Ask women to fill in their handouts, allowing plenty of time.

2   Get the group to brainstorm onto flipchart paper some issues in each area ('Getting here', 'Taking part' and 'As black women'). Keep this paper – it will act as a reminder for the group.

Discussion
Discuss some of the following issues (if relevant) with the group.

1   What does 'taking part' in a group actually mean to us?

2 Why might black women not come along to or take part in groups/meetings?

3 What past experiences of groups do we have? Were there difficulties in getting there and taking part?

4 How can we tackle these issues in this group?

10A Getting here, taking part, as black women

1 Tick any of the following issues which are relevant to you and your group.

2 How could you deal with them in a positive way?

Getting here

Employers not seeing my involvement as a priority, or making me take annual leave.

Other demands on my time.

A lot to do in a fairly short time: expectations too great.

Sickness and ill-health – perhaps reflecting the stresses in black women's lives.

Not being able to stay all day or for all of the meeting.

Access for women with special needs.

Disability transport being unreliable and time-consuming – a meeting can mean a day out.

Any others?

Taking part

Difficulty in relating the course/group to my experiences.

Don't understand/agree with the language and methods being used.

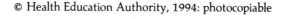

Difficulty with other people's attitude towards me when I'm here.

Not clear about my role in the group.

Feel unsure about sharing information about myself with this particular group.

If other people seem confident, will I end up feeling unable to make my own decisions?

Different priorities for my own time.

Any others?

As a group of black women

Fear of dragging ourselves down with differences and conflicts as a group.

Fears about being seen as different from others ('not being black enough').

Will I be rejected by my community?

Not being able to be assertive with each other.

Any others?

11 Ground rules

It is important to have positive ways of working together in groups so that differences and conflict don't end up destroying the group or get in the way of what the group is about. We can do this by having basic guidelines or ground rules.

11A Thinking about ground rules

EXERCISE

Purpose
To understand the role of ground rules.

Suitable for
A new group unfamiliar with ground rules.

Materials
Copies of handout 11A for each woman.

Method
Explain that this exercise is about the role of ground rules, not about developing them at this stage. Ask women to read the handout. Then, in either small groups, or one large one, ask them to think about and discuss the questions.

Discussion
In the main group, discuss how women would like to develop ground rules. Would they like to agree their own, or work from a basic set of rules which other women have found useful?

11B Developing ground rules

EXERCISE

Purpose
To develop ground rules to promote positive working in groups.

Suitable for
A new group.

Materials

Flipchart paper, marker pens.

For variation: as above, plus a copy of handouts 11B and 11C, and pens for each woman.

Method

1 If the group wants to develop its own ground rules from scratch, brainstorm ideas onto flipchart paper. You might want to consider:

   - language

   - differences and judgements

   - respect

   - confidentiality

2 From these, agree some clear ground rules for the group.

Variation

1 Give out copies of the two handouts.

2 Get women to fill them in individually or in small groups, and then feed back their views to the main group.

3 Use these to agree some clear ground rules, and write them on the flipchart.

Discussion

Discuss the ground rules developed, making sure all women agree with them. Stress that ground rules are about negotiation, and in relation to health and well-being they can provide us with a way of communicating with others that involves respect and co-operation. You could display the agreed ground rules during future sessions.

11A Using ground rules

Some of the things women have said about ground rules

- If ground rules are defined for us beforehand, without our participation, they can have less value.

- Groups with a history – established groups or social (friendship) groups – have patterns of their own.

- People have to want to work together.

- Sometimes ground rules do not acknowledge existing conflicts.

- We need to spend time on ground rules to make sure that all women feel included and get involved.

- We need to use language that we understand when defining ground rules.

- Ground rules are about trying to create a positive way of working together.

- Ground rules are for identifying the group's task. They make us define (and perhaps change) the nature of the group.

Questions

1 What do you know about ground rules in groups?

2 How do you feel about using them?

3 Would you like to have them worked out in advance or get this group to agree some?

4 How can we make them work in this group?

11B Blocks

The following are blocks which may cause disharmony in the group.

- Stereotyping each other

- Using confusing language

- Making assumptions (about sexuality, background, etc.)

- Treating the black community as if we are all the same

- Projecting or generalising – saying 'we' when we mean 'I'

1 Tick the ones you agree with and explain why.

2 Cross the ones you disagree with and explain why.

3 Add any other points in the space below:

11C Bridges

The following list includes attitudes and behaviours that may enable us to work productively and realistically, have fun and feel safe in the group.

- Taking responsibility for our own learning

- Challenging opinions

- Accepting others' differences or points of view

- Being non-judgemental

- Being accountable to group members: sharing information we feel safe with

- Acknowledging mistakes and dealing with them constructively

- Being specific

- Maintaining confidentiality

1 Tick the ones you agree with and explain why.
2 Cross the ones you have difficulty with and explain why.
3 Add any other points in the space below:

12 Working together

The following exercises look at ways of working together as a group, and issues that may come up for group members. The exercises can be useful for established groups, where women know each other, but may not have had an opportunity to acknowledge what they need or want from each other.

12A Warm-up around differences

EXERCISE

Purpose
To enable groups to share their differences and similarities.

Suitable for
A new group.

Materials
A large map of the world, cards with flags, emblems or names of different countries on them, and coloured stickers. (Try to ensure you have an up-to-date map.)

Either think beforehand about which countries are likely to come up, or get women to put cards on countries as part of a group activity.

Method
1   Give each woman a set of stickers of the same colour.

2   Ask women to take turns introducing themselves through their country of origin or birthplace and then to identify countries which mean something to them by placing a sticker on each.

3   Encourage them to talk a little about their connections with these countries – through families, friendships and so on.

Discussion
Ask the group to discuss what this exercise has brought up for them. Had women made assumptions about others' countries of origin or experiences? How much do these things say about us? What are their implications for women working together?

12B How do we relate to each other as black women?

E X E R C I S E

Purpose

- To explore some of the difficulties in working with differences between black women.

- To find ways of addressing these difficulties and to promote healthier relationships.

Suitable for

A new group.

Materials

A copy of handout 12A for each woman.

Method

1 Ask women to read the handout.

2 In small groups, talk about the points it raises.

Discussion

In the main group, encourage women to discuss the following issues:

- Do you agree with what the handout is saying?

- Do you find it difficult to express differences with other black women? Why? How do you deal with these differences?

- What are these difficulties and differences about?

Ask women to think of a particular example where black women have to deal with differences between themselves (perhaps if one woman is a health professional, another her patient; or where one woman identifies as 'black', another as 'Asian'). Get the group to discuss this with the following questions in mind:

- How do you feel in this situation? Why?

- Does it depend on who the other black women are? Why? Would the situation change if a white person were present?

- Are these positive ways of dealing with disagreements?

- Can you think of any 'more positive ways' to deal with differences in similar situations?

Round off the discussion with a summary of the main points raised and their health implications.

12C Positive ways of relating to each other

EXERCISE

Purpose
- To distinguish between criticism and constructive feedback.
- To encourage constructive feedback.

Suitable for
A group that has built up a level of trust.

Materials
A copy of handout 12B for each woman. Two large sheets of paper. Pens.

Method
1   Ask women to read the handout.

2   Split the group into two. Give each group a large piece of paper. Ask one group to think about (and write down) what they understand 'criticism' to mean, and the other to think about what is meant by 'constructive feedback'. What is the purpose of each? What effect might they have on health?

3   In the main group, ask someone from each group to summarise their findings.

Discussion
- Is it useful to distinguish between criticism and constructive feedback? Why?
- Does our willingness to accept and give feedback depend on who's involved? Why?
- What helps women to receive and give feedback to others?

12D Who do you trust? You can't tell nobody anything!

EXERCISE

Purpose
- To explore blocks to trust and confidentiality in black women's groups.
- To help women work out for ourselves what trust means.
- To work towards developing trust to promote well-being in the group.

Suitable for
Later in the group's life, or an established group (perhaps before looking at sexual health).

Materials

A copy of handout 12C for each woman.

Method

1 Give out copies of the handout.

2 Get women to discuss the handout in groups of about four.

3 Share the following questions between the groups.

- What do the statements in the handout mean to you?

- Are there any you would add, change or take away?

- Are these barriers *your* barriers to trust?

- Do you have any particular 'blocks' about trust in this group? What are they? How do they affect health and well-being?

- What do we mean by trust?

- Why is it important to us?

- What leads us to trust others?

- How can we – as a group – take responsibility for being trusted?

- What will enable each group member to ask for what she wants:

  - from other women here?

  - elsewhere?

Discussion

Back in the main group, encourage women from each small group to feed back what they have come up with. How can this group use the points noted to enable trust to grow? What are the implications of this kind of trust for our health and well-being?

12E How do others see me? How do I see myself?

EXERCISE

Purpose

To explore the way we stereotype people.

Suitable for

A group where trust and support have been established.

Materials

None.

Method

1 Ask women to find a partner they don't know and sit opposite her.

2 Women then take it in turns to observe their partner carefully for three minutes. Ask women to look at each other as if for the first time without making judgements based on what they know or assume. What can they tell about women from what they're wearing, their facial expressions, or how they hold their bodies?

3 Each woman then tells her partner what she sees, and her partner talks about how this fits in with her own perceptions of herself.

Discussion

Back in the main group, get women to discuss the following questions:

- What did you see? How accurate were you? Did you fall into the trap of making assumptions?

- Did you find it difficult to state what you saw? Did you feel you had to be polite? How honest were you able to be about your observations on dress, hairstyle, hair texture, skin tone, identity marks, posture? Why?

- What do these physical characteristics signify to the observer? How accurately do they fit how we see ourselves?

- Discuss how you might interpret your observations – being heavily built and wearing spectacles equals strong and studious, for example.

- How do your first impressions of someone affect your response to her?

- How did you feel about someone describing you? How did you feel about her getting you right or wrong?

You could then lead on to a discussion about the kinds of assumptions and stereotypes we use every day when dealing with people. How might these ways of seeing help or hinder working with other black women? What implications might they have for our health and well-being?

12A Relating to each other as black women

Everyday life is often full of conflicts about views, values and opinions. Many of us can find it very difficult to express differences with other black women – to be assertive with each other.

We might have fears and anxieties about saying the wrong thing, offending others, showing ignorance, being rejected, or viewed as not being 'black enough'; or we may just want to keep the peace.

It's useful to explore what these fears are about and find ways of expressing ourselves in the group, based on co-operation and mutual respect – fostering a healthier relationship with others.

It can sometimes help to view our differences as a way of asserting or expressing ourselves as individuals – illustrating the diversity there is amongst us, rather than allowing it to get in the way of us working together positively.

12B Feedback

Giving feedback to each other as black women is an important way of acknowledging and supporting each other's contribution in the group and elsewhere in a health-enhancing way.

It is also something we can all benefit from: recognising and honouring diversity can help us to deal much more productively with other people.

Considering how we do this helps us to assess how we support others and to look at our own response to feedback from others.

We can also look closely at how we approach others over difference: what are our own strategies for raising issues or concerns? Do we tend to criticise women who hold views different from our own? Is it possible to separate someone's ideas from her as a person?

Handout 12B

12C Trust

Trust is an important ingredient in any healthy relationship –
with health professionals, our families, or our friends, for
example. It is based on mutual respect and co-operation.

Our difficulties with trust may be based on:

- believing that we alone know how to support ourselves;

- believing we can't trust anyone enough to ask for and get
  support;

- being afraid of exposing ourselves (particularly our
  weaknesses) to other black people; being seen as vulnerable
  and not living up to others' expectations;

- being afraid of rejection by people we care about.

13 Assertiveness and our own health

It is important for facilitators to appreciate the difficulty that many black women have with assertiveness, health and sexual health. 'Assertiveness' may suggest ways of acquiring skills and modes of behaviour that some black women are not comfortable with or do not feel are relevant to them. Other women say that they do not feel assertiveness takes into account the social, environmental and cultural influences on their lives – factors which can limit their ability to promote their own health. For some, sexual health and women's health issues are taboo areas.

We need to acknowledge these concerns. They can prevent women from seeking and getting help from each other in the group or elsewhere.

The first two exercises in this section are about identifying these concerns, and may be useful with groups which are sceptical about what 'assertiveness' can offer them. They can also help refine and renegotiate what women mean by 'assertiveness' – enabling groups to come up with their own workable definitions.

The remaining exercises tackle how to apply ideas of assertiveness to women's lives.

13A What's it all about for me?

EXERCISE

Purpose
To identify difficulties women experience in understanding 'assertiveness' and its relevance to them.

Suitable for
A group which hasn't yet defined assertiveness or assessed its usefulness.

Materials
Flipchart paper, marker pen.

Method
1   Ask women to say whether they experience difficulty in making sense of assertiveness and relating it to their health and sexual health. Why is this? (You may want to make

some suggestions – language, meaning, relevance, taboos, and so on.)

2 Write these difficulties up on the flipchart.

3 How would women in the group like to look at these difficulties? They may want to:

- de-mystify assertiveness

- relate assertiveness to themselves and their health

- address why they need to look at sexual health

- work through any taboos around sexual health.

Discussion

Summarise the main points and health issues raised. Can the group reach a consensus on what they would like to look at? Facilitators should then choose appropriate exercises from this section to use next.

13B Making connections

EXERCISE

Purpose

To identify and begin to work through difficulties women experience in understanding 'assertiveness' and its relevance to them.

Suitable for

A group which hasn't worked out how it feels about assertiveness, particularly if women are experiencing difficulties in coming up with ideas of their own.

Materials

A copy of handouts 13A and 13B for each woman, pens.

Method

Ask women to fill in the handouts, either alone or in small groups.

Discussion

In the main group, discuss the following points:

- How do the issues raised in the handouts affect our health and well-being?

- How would group members suggest dealing with these issues in a positive way?
- Is there an obvious way forward for the group?

13C Thoughts about assertiveness

EXERCISE

Purpose
To explore women's feelings and views about assertiveness and to think about positive ways of using it.

Suitable for
A new group which has cleared up any preconceptions about assertiveness and is ready to look at it more closely.

Materials
A copy of handouts 13C and 13D for each woman, pens.

Method
Ask women to fill in handout 13C without discussing it at this point. Explain that the exercise is not about having the right or wrong answers, but about giving group members the opportunity to find out how they feel about assertiveness.

Discussion
Discuss women's responses, using the following prompts:

- What did you think of the statements?
- Could you relate to them?
- Why did you respond the way you did?

Finally, give out copies of handout 13D, and go through the checklist. Ask women for their feedback on the exercise as a whole.

13D The implications of assertiveness

EXERCISE

Purpose
To help women define how assertiveness relates to health.

Suitable for
Women who are comfortable using the term 'assertiveness'. It is important to highlight that respect for other people's rights is central to assertive behaviour.

Materials

A copy of handout 13E for each woman, pens.

Method

Ask women to fill in the handout, either singly or in small groups.

Discussion

In the main group, discuss the following points.

- Do these definitions mean anything to you? Why?

- How do these issues affect your health? Can you give examples from your own experience? (For example, does talking to your doctor about your health, or making a complaint about a service, affect your confidence?) What would enable you to deal with these situations more effectively?

- Which statements are meaningful, and which aren't? What would you add, remove, or change; and why?

13E Thoughts about sexual health

E X E R C I S E

Purpose

To explore women's feelings and views about sexual health.

Suitable for

A group that has established trust.

Materials

A copy of handout 13F for each woman.

Method

As for *Thoughts about assertiveness* (exercise 13C).

Discussion

As for *Thoughts about assertiveness*, adding the following discussion points to the three there.

1 Which statements do we think are about promoting our health and well-being as women? Why?

2   Which ones are not? Why not? You might want to discuss
     with the group other ways to:

- work positively in relationships to promote well-being;

- feel positive about our health in relation to our bodies;

- look after our own health and well-being, and support
     others in looking after theirs.

13A Assertiveness: difficulties

The following three lists are negative ways of seeing assertiveness, health and sexual health in relation to ourselves.

1   Tick the statements you agree with and explain why.

2   Cross the statements you don't agree with and explain why.

3   Add any other points.

Difficulties with assertiveness

- It presents us with images we cannot relate to – white middle-class images from books, perhaps.

- It's about telling someone what to do or how to behave in certain situations.

- It doesn't include our language, culture, way of expressing ourselves and different experiences, particularly in relation to health.

- Black women are not recognised as being assertive! They are often seen as either aggressive or submissive.

- Racism affects black women's health and ability to be assertive: having constantly to react to it or actively combat it.

- It lacks a perspective for black women – who we are, where we are now and where we are going (as individuals and as communities).

- Other points:

Barriers to achieving health

- Believing the negative messages and images presented to us about black people generally (internalising racism).

- Being silenced by others.

- Feeling vulnerable.

- Having to deal with contradictory feelings and messages.

- Not having the know-how.

- Lacking confidence.

- Other points:

Difficulties with sexual health

- Cultural taboos.

- It's personal.

- Anxieties and concerns around assumptions, stereotypes.

- Confidentiality issues.

- Other points:

13B Assertiveness: opportunities

The following two lists are positive ways of linking assertiveness, health and sexual health and finding them useful to ourselves.

1   Tick the suggestions you agree with and explain why.

2   Cross the suggestions you disagree with and explain why.

3   Add any other points.

Ways forward

- We need to build confidence in ourselves and relate assertiveness, health and sexual health to our lives and experiences.

- We need to value our resources and share them with others to promote health and well-being.

- We need to develop our awareness of what we do and why in the difficult situations we face with others, and how our responses can affect our health.

- We need to work out how we see our well-being and ability to be assertive now. We can look at: this group, work-related issues, home, and so on.

- We need to recognise the encouragement and support we give, get and can ask for which will enable us and others to move forward with ourselves, our lives and health.

- Other points:

Some strategies

- Finding ways of exploring the choices we are able to make – and what limits them.

- Using opportunities to talk and get support.

- Expressing anger and other emotions in a healthy way and finding ways of channelling them into positive action rather than repressing them, or allowing them to be destructive.

- Looking beyond individual remedies to group approaches where women can agree a way forward.

- Sharing our experiences with each other; validating our own and others' experiences.

- Working on taboo areas – sexual health and its implications for women's health, perhaps.

- Negotiating and communicating with other women.

- Moving away from images of ourselves that frustrate growth and personal development; not getting stuck, or reduced to self-pity or bitterness.

- Other points:

13C What I feel about assertiveness

The following are some views which have been expressed by black women about assertiveness. Mark 'A' for agree; 'D' for disagree; and 'N' for neutral.

1   It's white and middle-class.

2   You've got to say things in a certain way.

3   Black women are already assertive and strong. They have to be.

4   It's not nice to criticise people. Some people can't help the way they are.

5   You get into too much trouble.

6   It's aggressive.

7   I can never make up my mind what I want to do, so it's not my thing.

8   Some people have got it, some people ain't.

9   It's not for people who want a quiet life.

10   It takes a lot of energy and courage.

11   It's about people's attitude towards me and how I deal with them.

12   You've got to be prepared to listen to the other person. Everyone has their point of view.

13   It's about the strength we can have when we come together as black women.

14   It's about finding me.

13D What is assertiveness?

1   Self-expressive – how we express ourselves.

2   Respectful of other people's rights.

3   Honest.

4   Direct and firm.

5   Promoting equality and benefiting both sides in a relationship.

6   Talking and communicating information – feelings, rights, facts, opinions, beliefs, requests and limits.

7   Communicating clearly – not necessarily talking but also active listening, signing, gestures, eye-contact, using face and whole body, and timing.

8   Appropriate for the person and the situation.

9   Socially responsible.

10 Something which is learnt (you're not born with it).

Adapted from *Your perfect right* (Impact)

13E Defining assertiveness

The following definitions of assertiveness have been developed by a group of black women.

1   Tick the definitions you agree with and explain why.

2   Cross the definitions you disagree with and explain why.

3   Add any other points.

What does assertiveness mean to me?

- Having strategies to deal with other people's attitudes to me.

- Being able to do and think what feels comfortable.

- Having no regrets.

- Taking risks.

- Going against the grain – sometimes against the black community.

- Finding me.

- Dealing with the pain put on me by my community.

- Being able to recognise and challenge hidden agendas.

- Having choices, using opportunities.

- Other points:

What does assertiveness mean to us as group members?

- Collective strength.

- Having the confidence to say what we mean in situations where we don't feel supported – in situations with white people, perhaps.

- Recognising that our cultures are not static – and working out what we can do to change and develop them.

- Challenging stereotypes which label black women as weaker than black men.

- Recognising and building on the strengths we have as black women.
- Defining ourselves as we choose; finding our own identities.
- Other points:

What stops me from being assertive?

- People not listening.
- Feeling patronised.
- Being ignored.
- Isolation.
- Being stereotyped by our language, clothing, culture, and so on.
- Fear of rejection.
- Not being black (Asian/Chinese . . .) enough.
- Other points:

What enables me to be assertive?

- Being able to share specific experiences with other black women.
- Participating, and being able to raise issues.
- Providing role models for others.
- Challenging negative stereotypes and images.
- Knowing who I am, valuing myself, and being clear about what I want and what my limitations are.
- Respecting other people.
- Having access to information and support.
- Not being motivated by guilt.
- Having a sense of a strong black community and a black community health agenda.
- Other points:

13F What I feel about sexual health

The following are some views which have been expressed by black women about sexual health. Mark 'A' for agree; 'D' for disagree; and 'N' for neutral.

- What people do behind closed doors is their own business.
- What's all the fuss about?
- There's little information or guidance to see you through.
- It's about exploring and expressing your own sexuality.
- On sexual attraction: it's not how you look, it's what you're like.
- On body image and confidence: it's about reducing my weight so I look good.
- On breastfeeding: it's all right in private, but not in public.
- On sexual relationships: it's about feeling good and having a good time.
- On sex: mixed feelings, feeling vulnerable, wanting to be loved, feeling used.
- On safer sex: finding ways of avoiding unwanted sex is safer sex!
- On expressing oneself sexually: if you're out for a good time or are a good-time girl, you're slack!
- The biggest barrier to women asserting themselves is other women – their mothers, sisters, aunts, mothers-in-law, neighbours and so-called friends!
- Not feeling pressured into having sex or a particular type of sex which you don't want.
- Enjoying sex, without disapproval.

14 Speaking out: weighing up the costs to health

The following exercises look at the dilemmas many women confront when speaking out about issues that are important to their health. One way forward is to look at how to weigh up the health costs (emotional, sexual, physical and so on) of such assertiveness. Knowing the risks and opportunities can sometimes give us the courage we need; and understanding the context of our own decisions can enable us to begin to make choices.

14A Raising the issues

EXERCISE

Purpose
- To identify and work through the dilemmas we face when protecting our own health and well-being or helping others to do the same.
- To share ways of dealing with taboo subjects.

Suitable for
An established or supportive group.

Materials
A copy of handout 14A for all participants. Examples of appropriate stories from the media – problem pages from the black press, for example.

Method
1 Ask women to read the handout.
2 Get the group to decide on one or two issues to look at which they feel are relevant to them.

Discussion
- What anxieties or concerns do we have about considering taboo subjects?
- Is there a fear that if we speak out about these issues, we

may be labelled 'not black enough'? (Maybe people think that we have been duped by others – perhaps white people – into undermining our communities?)

● Are we frightened of being rejected by our families and friends, and not belonging anywhere?

● What are the costs to our own health or that of others when we take no action?

● How can we support each other as individuals or as a group to be assertive on our own terms?

● Are there any media examples of situations where others have had similar dilemmas to face (for example, the 1991 Anita Hill/Clarence Thomas case in the USA)?

14B Thinking about female circumcision

EXERCISE

Purpose

To understand the dilemmas some women face about the culture and practice of female circumcision.

Suitable for

A group where a good level of trust has been developed, and which has covered the previous exercise, *Raising the issues*.

Materials

A copy of handout 14B for each woman. You could also think about preparing your own background sheet about female circumcision, perhaps using some of the resources at the end of this book. You may want to include the various types of circumcision performed; where and why it is practised; and the law relating to female circumcision. The London Black Women's Health Action Project can supply a book and video (both called *Silent tears*) which you might want to use with the group.

Method

1   Divide women into two groups and give them each a copy of the handout.

2   In the groups, ask them to look at the statements and discuss them.

Discussion

Ask the small groups to feed back their discussions. Recap and summarise the main points. (You could complete the session by showing the video, *Silent Tears*.)

14C Some things just are!

E X E R C I S E

Purpose
To look at why women might resign themselves to accepting things.

Suitable for
A group that is trusting and supportive, as a follow-on from the previous exercise. This exercise may need careful facilitation to ensure that women feel they are in an unthreatening and positive environment.

Materials
A copy of handout 14C for each woman.

Method
Ask women to read through the handout.

Discussion
- What does the expression 'Some things just are' mean to you? (Women may want to discuss resigning themselves, giving up, or passively accepting things they are not happy with.)

- Can you think of some things you believe 'just are' in black women's lives? (You might want to focus on the examples given – adding to them, removing ones the group doesn't agree with.)

- Are there any benefits to this particular outlook – handing down and preserving values, perhaps (sometimes an effective survival strategy)?

- What are the limitations of this outlook? How do these affect your health? Who benefits from you adopting this position?

- What are the ways of moving forward when you are stuck or unable to see a way of helping yourself to health and well-being? Can a group approach help?

Draw together the main points raised.

14D Influences on our sexual health

E X E R C I S E

Purpose

To enable women to share their experiences of growing up and the influences on their sexual health in a supportive group.

Suitable for

A group that has developed trust. The exercise divides into three parts (early experiences; information and support; dealing with contradictions) which can follow one another, although not necessarily in the same session.

Materials

A copy of handouts 14D, 14E and 14F for each woman. Encourage group members to bring in early photographs of themselves and their families.

Method

1   Divide women into small groups.

2   Ask women to read the handouts and discuss the issues they raise. Encourage them to tell their own stories and to listen to each other.

Discussion

In the main group, get women to feed back on what the exercise has raised for them about their own sexual or emotional journeys. Do they feel that there are now things that they have become aware of (attitudes, behaviour patterns, assumptions) which they might like to reconsider?

14A Staying silent

Our needs as black women can sometimes be at odds with those of our communities. Many of us face dilemmas when we try to promote our health or support others to promote theirs. But sometimes it can help to look carefully at exactly what the risks are of speaking out. Often, to protect our own health in an assertive way we need to know what will happen to us and the burden we will have to bear if we challenge practices, attitudes and behaviour that adversely affect us or other women in our communities.

The following have raised dilemmas for a number of women in the past:

- Female 'circumcision' (clitoridectomy)

- Domestic violence

- Child abuse/incest

- Sexual harassment

- Homophobia

- Attitudes to HIV and AIDS

14B Female circumcision

If we have no direct contact with women who have undergone female circumcision, it can be difficult to understand the enormous pressure on some women to comply with the practice, or equally to understand how some women may unquestioningly have their daughters circumcised.

The statements below describe black women's experiences of female circumcision.

- What are the dilemmas or issues behind these statements?
- Can you relate to any of these statements?
- How would you deal with similar situations or reactions?
- How would you support others in this or a similar situation?

1   Nawal says that it was the turning point in her life. 'The circumcision either makes you really angry or one becomes so passive that one continues in the role mapped out. It is another form of construction. Women are constructed for reproduction and man's pleasure. Her whole life is planned. From birth to death – it's settled.'

2   'They still see it as an essential part of socialisation in Somali culture. They just don't see it as a problem. It is a problem. It causes pain. It is debilitating. One woman I talked to was for it. But by the end you could see that she saw the contradictions. She said "if I had an education like you I would be against it, but I don't have an education. I can't get a job so I have to comply", meaning "if I wasn't dependent, if I could support myself, I would". I "need" to belong to my community.'

3   'I think it is a bad thing really. Both my daughters were done. It was my family's will. It was just done somehow. No discussion. It just is.'

4   'I don't want to talk about this [sex and sexuality]. We don't talk about these things. It was very bad. People would not understand. Nobody talks about these things. I always had problems with my blood and things. Nobody thinks it is connected to the circumcision. I was very frightened when it was done and have always problems and fear.'

▶

© Health Education Authority, 1994: photocopiable

5 'Now that circumcision is becoming a public issue, women feel people are trespassing and interfering because it's about themselves, it's a private thing. They probably think that nothing happens to anyone else. Circumcision causes bad health, bad childbirth, bad sex . . . If women want satisfaction then they have to stop circumcision.'

6 [Author] The real problem is how to maintain certain traditions and rituals which are positive and central to all the community and eliminate others which are harmful: to make [sure] the people behind the 'decision' need not feel the loss of their roots and culture, but just accept recognition of the harmful aspects. Certainly a comparative tool (a study which is being undertaken at the moment) could be useful at least to point out that in nearly all societies, as far as women are concerned, some harmful practices were and are undertaken, even in the so-called civilised societies.

From *Silent tears* (London Black Women's Health Action Project)

14C Some things just are!

Our list of some things that 'just are' might include:

- the grind of daily life
- just coping and surviving
- lurching from crisis to crisis.

These might be based on our own beliefs or a real experience:

- it is unsafe to walk the streets at night
- all men are the same and out for one thing
- men speak on behalf of the family or community
- discrimination and inequality are facts of life
- it is impossible to challenge the status quo.

It can be difficult to stand back and look at ourselves and our ways of behaving and thinking and their effect on our health, self-esteem and relationships with others. Acknowledging the health effects of thinking that 'some things just are' can be an important starting point in learning more about ourselves.

Handout 14C

14D Early experiences

1 Which women featured prominently in your life when you were growing up – mothers, sisters, aunts, grandmothers, great-aunts?

2 How were they viewed by other people? Why?

3 What kind of role models did they provide you with in terms of: their attitudes to their own and others' bodies; how they looked after themselves; their relationships with other people (particularly men)?

4 How did they influence you?

5 How did those influences affect you at the time?

6 How do you see them now?

14E Information and support

1　At the time, how did you experience and understand puberty/your first period and the changes in your body?

2　What information were you given about:

● 　the changes in your body, and how to look after it?

● 　marriage, sex, babies?

3　How do you go about getting the information and support you need regarding health checks (screenings), health scares and your own health concerns?

4　How do you bring up health matters with your daughters, sisters, nieces, and friends? Do you feel able to give information and support about sex, sexual feelings, relationships, sexuality, and sexually transmitted diseases (including HIV)? Do you have any blocks about these kinds of conversations? How would you go about addressing these issues and blocks in an assertive way?

© Health Education Authority, 1994: photocopiable

14F Dealing with contradictions

1   What images of women and our sexualities are presented:
    - in the media?

    - in films made by or directed at our communities?

    - in advertising?

    - through religious or cultural teachings?

2   What are the contradictions between what you are like and how other people think women should be?

3   How do you go about resolving these contradictions?

15 Counteracting the stresses in our lives

When we are not able to influence the inequalities we meet daily, we have to find our own ways of counteracting their effects on our health and self-esteem. The following exercises should enable you to help group members recognise and value the various sources of strength, support and encouragement they already have or can develop.

15A What is the black community?

EXERCISE

Purpose
To explore what 'the black community' means for black women; how they relate to the black community; and how this relationship may affect their health and well-being.

Suitable for
A new group.

Materials
None.

Method
Use the following questions to facilitate a group discussion.

Discussion
- What do we mean by 'community'? (It may be useful to look at the different ways in which the word is used: community care, community association, community centre, community work, community worker.)

- Is there a black community? How do you see it? Do you feel part of it? Do you think you should?

- What are the benefits to our health and well-being of being part of a community?

- What are the stresses of being part of a community (particularly a close-knit community)? How do we deal with them?

- What does this say about us as a group of black women?

15B Black and feelings of – pride, unease or indifference?

E X E R C I S E

Purpose

To enable group members to begin to explore feelings and images they have about themselves as black women.

Suitable for

A group with a good level of trust. (Groups at a stage where they want to look at issues of self-definition, self-acceptance and similarities and differences between group members. It may have particular relevance for young women.)

Materials

A copy of handout 15A for each woman. You may want to rewrite it, replacing 'black' with whichever term women prefer to define themselves (their nationality or country of origin, or specific ethnic grouping, perhaps).

Method

Ask women to read the handout.

Discussion

Discuss the following questions with the group, adapting them if need be.

- Do you identify as a black woman? What does it mean to you?

- How comfortable do you feel in relation to:
  - Other black women? Why?
  - Black men? Why?
  - White people? Why?

- Is how you define yourself important to you? Why?

- Are there labels which others apply to you which you reject? Why?

- How do you tell people what (if anything) you would like to be called?

- Did members of the group have different answers to the two previous questions? Why? What does that tell us about ourselves as a group?

- How can we work with these differences?

- What are the health implications of defining ourselves in certain ways?

To close the exercise, recap the main points.

15C Black women: saying what we want to say

E X E R C I S E

Purpose

- To look at the difficulties some black women face in asserting themselves in relation to those (especially white people) in authority.

- To try to draw out issues of power and racism and to look at their effect on black women's confidence, relationships, and emotional health and well-being.

Suitable for

Groups in which a level of trust has been developed.

Materials

None.

Method

Facilitate a group discussion using the following questions. (You may need to clarify points and illustrate with examples of your own.)

Discussion

- Why do some black women find it difficult to asert themselves in situations with white people on their own terms, even if the discussion is about their own needs?

- Can anybody think of a situation where this has happened to her (at work or with a health professional, perhaps)? What stopped you from speaking up? What would have enabled you to speak up? Are there any strategies you can use to feel more confident next time?

- How can black women deal with officialdom if their spoken English is used to undermine their self-confidence? What strategies can be used in this type of situation? Which are most effective?

- Why do black women sometimes feel they have to comply with other people's demands and ways of doing things? How do these issues affect their personal health and well-being and that of their communities?

Close the exercise by recapping the main points and any conclusions the group may have come to.

15D Sometimes it's hard to say no

E X E R C I S E

Purpose
To explore difficulties in setting boundaries and saying no; and to address their effect on black women's health and well-being.

Suitable for
Groups who have established a good level of trust.

Materials
A copy of handout 15B for each woman.

Method
Ask women to read the handout.

Discussion
Facilitate a group discussion based on the following questions:

- Does the handout describe something you can relate to? Do you have examples of situations in which you have found it hard to say no? How have you dealt with these situations?

- What implications does not being able to say no have for black women's health and well-being?

- What are the difficulties in saying no to:
    - in-laws/families?
    - communities?
    - workers/employers?

- Do black women need to be supported in order to say no? Where can that support be found?

- What are the main ways of setting realistic boundaries? (Recognising that we have rights; finding ways of dealing positively with our feelings of guilt, and so on.)

Close the discussion by recapping and summarising the main points.

15E Valuing the support we give and receive

E X E R C I S E

Purpose

To encourage women to look at what support means to them and the role it can play in improving health and well-being in their lives.

Suitable for

Early on in a group's life.

Materials

None.

Method

Discuss what 'support' means to the group, adapting and using some or all of the following questions. You might want to distinguish between support which encourages or builds confidence (empowers women to deal with stresses and difficulties in their lives) and support which does not. Encourage women to be specific in their responses to the questions and to give examples.

Discussion

- In what ways do women give support to others in the community? (Community health work, supporting family members, being involved with church, temple, mosque, perhaps.)

- Who values the work and support women give? In what way?

- How do women value their own work?

- What do we mean by support? (What do others ask of us?) What do we actually give or get when we ask for support for ourselves?

- Why is it sometimes difficult to ask for support from others?

- How do we go about giving support to each other in this group?

- How important is support to health and well-being?

- How can we help ourselves when what people offer is not what we want? (You may need to illustrate this point with an example.)

Close the exercise by highlighting issues that have come up in the discussion.

15A Defining ourselves

The general feelings we have about ourselves as black women can affect how we see ourselves. These feelings may be ones of confidence and pride, or unease and indifference. They can also have an impact on our self-confidence and emotional health and well-being when we deal with people – other black women, black men and white people.

Some of us find defining ourselves as black an important expression of our identity; this says something about how we want to be regarded by others. External appearances can help to send out this message. We might express our individuality and culture through the clothes or jewellery we wear, how we style our hair or the way we cover our heads.

Other women's experiences of stereotyping and labelling lead them to feel that identifying themselves too closely with a particular group can limit their own sense of themselves – and others' perceptions of them.

15B Saying no

Some of us find it difficult to separate out our own needs and identity from those of others – particularly our families and communities.

Our sense of self can get lost in the different and sometimes conflicting roles and responsibilities we carry as partners, wives, daughters-in-law, mothers, sisters and workers (particularly for those of us working with our own communities).

We may, for example, find it hard to manage the many demands made on us by our community and jobs. We may feel overburdened and ultimately responsible for meeting these demands, particularly when there is no one else to meet them – if we are the only worker with language skills, for example.

This situation can often be complicated by conflicting and sometimes unrealistic expectations placed on us by our bosses or other workers.

16 Case studies: supporting others

The following exercises are case studies based on real situations. In the first, told by the woman's counsellor, personal details have been changed so that the woman remains anonymous. The second represents the experience of Jacky Downer, which she uses to stimulate discussion about self-advocacy issues for black people with learning difficulties.

These case studies can give facilitators models for discussion, which can help women to learn about others' needs. From this, you can look at how group members might begin to offer support to one another and others.

16A Case studies

EXERCISE

Purpose
To explore ways of supporting others.

Suitable for
Any stage of a group.

Materials
A copy of handouts 16A and 16B for each woman. (Or you might feel it's more appropriate to just cover one of the case studies.)

Method
1   Ask women to read and discuss the handout(s) in small groups, noting down their responses to the questions.

2   In the main group, get small groups to feed back what they have been discussing.

Discussion
Finish off by recapping the main issues.

(Many thanks to Jacky Downer for providing the Project with material for handout 16B.)

16A Sharma's dilemma

The situation

Sharma was taking tablets which the consultant had prescribed for her depression. She telephoned the centre to tell me that she was afraid. The nurses and doctor were telling her she would have to keep taking medication or else she would end up in hospital again.

Sharma's main concern was that she was expecting a baby and that she was taking substances into her body that were not making her feel any better and might be harmful to her baby.

'I want to breastfeed my baby. What am I to do? They say it's not advisable to breastfeed while I am on medication.'

The counsellor's response

I told Sharma that she had a right to choose whether to breastfeed or not, and that this should be her starting point. Once the choice was made, the effects of medication had to be considered.

'It is your right to decide to stop taking medication because you want to breastfeed. If you choose to do this, you must let your doctor know. You must request advice and support to stop the medication. Do not just stop, as you may suffer withdrawal symptoms and need a lot of support. Support is available and there are many organisations that offer counselling support.

Do seek help from these organisations both before and after the baby's born, especially at times when you feel anxious or afraid of becoming ill again.'

Note

It is not easy for women who are in need of mental health support to be recognised as assertive and having the right to choose their treatment.

Friends and relatives can make this time easier by recognising the needs of pregnant women on medication. Women themselves should start recognising the need for support, and make these decisions early in the pregnancy.

Questions

1   Can you relate to Sharma's experience? In what way?

2   What would you do if you were:
   - Sharma?
   - a relative?
   - a friend?

3   What did you think of the counsellor's response? Did she overlook anything?

4   Why is it difficult for women who are in need of mental health support to be recognised as assertive, as in this case?

5   What are your experiences of mental illness (with family members, friends, etc.)?

6   What are your own attitudes and feelings about mental health?

7   What are some of the difficulties women experience in supporting others with mental health problems? How might we begin to address them assertively?

16B Black self-advocacy – my experience of being black and having a learning difficulty

Primary school

At primary school, in the early 1970s, I had difficulties with my work but no extra help was offered to me. When I was about ten, a man came into school and gave me some tests. No one explained to me or my parents that this person was coming to see me or what it was for.

Secondary school

Next thing I knew I was sent to a special school. In the beginning I was the only black pupil in my class. I had difficulty keeping up with the work because spelling was difficult for me but I understood most of what I had to do. I felt very confused and ashamed at being put into this school and other children used to make fun of me on my way to that school.

As I was the only black pupil who was also having difficulties with my learning, I felt very isolated. I found myself wishing I was white so that I would be accepted by the teachers and other pupils who were all white. As I moved into other classes other black pupils joined me. I felt a lot better, but much of my self-confidence had already gone.

Barriers

Teachers did not expect too much of me. The books and lessons did not show anything positive about black people. It seemed as though we had never given anything to the world.

Self-advocacy

I was not fortunate enough to get on to a self-advocacy scheme. I had to push for myself when I left school. Most people didn't want to employ a black person with learning difficulties. I started a course at Brixton College and some tutors there offered me a lot of help and encouraged me to be more confident and to speak up for myself. I was directed to the other people who identified my learning strengths and weaknesses.

I had a long hard struggle to get to where I am now. The struggle goes on daily for all black people, especially those with different kinds of learning difficulties. People still try to abuse me but I feel that I have something positive to offer others like myself who want to speak out on all sorts of issues that affect them.

Jacky Downer, Brixton College, September 1990

Questions

1 What do you think about Jacky's experiences?

2 Do they relate to your own experiences? In what ways?

3 What support would you have given as a parent, relative or friend to help Jacky deal with her issues and concerns? (Be specific.)

4 What do you think about people's rights to assert themselves as a parent, relative or child's guardian to safeguard the child's well-being?

5 What are the particular barriers black women with learning difficulties face in relation to their health and ability to assert themselves:

   • within their own community?

   • outside?

6 How can black women begin to address some of the barriers in an assertive way?

17 Activities to promote self-esteem and well-being

The following exercises are fun, flexible and will affirm the work the group has already done.

Both your own and the group's confidence in developing ideas on activities will depend on how you and the group want to define, understand or work with health, sexual health and assertiveness issues for yourselves.

Try to be imaginative and look at ways of adding to your own work materials from personal situations and events that are happening in your community, locally and nationally.

17A Stories

E X E R C I S E

Purpose
- To round off a session illustrating a theme or topic.
- To demonstrate ways of dealing with stressful or difficult situations or with taboo subjects.
- To inspire discussion.

Suitable for

Any stage in a group's life. Stories (whether we are telling our own or listening to other people's) can be an important way of validating women's experiences. Story-telling forms an integral part of handing down a community's culture.

Materials

In advance, you'll need to get the group to think about collecting examples of success stories from community newspapers, the national and local press, minority ethnic press, passages from autobiographies and from books women have at home. Encourage women to bring their own materials to ensure that you get a good spread which isn't limited to your own personal tastes and interests. You may also want to ensure that the stories represent as broad a spectrum of black women as possible, and that you use media which are accessible to people with various disabilities. Poetry, cartoons, pictures, photographs and sayings can also be used to tell a story or to illustrate important points.

Method

Ask women to introduce and present their stories, saying why they have chosen them.

Discussion

- Ask women what they thought of the stories.

- Get women to identify the strengths and personal resources of the main characters which enable them to deal with particular pressures. Is it their attitudes, thinking patterns, things they say to themselves or what they actually do which makes their stories useful?

- Could women see themselves using the same strategies or personal resources if they were in a similar situation? Would they use different ones? How would they go about supporting someone else in the same situation?

17B Activities

E X E R C I S E

Purpose

To enable women to share with each other: information, inspiration, education, discussion, recreation, relaxation and activities we enjoy and which promote our health, well-being and self-esteem. This could include going to see plays, group outings, celebrating festivals within our groups. Anything goes . . .

Suitable for

Any stage in a group's life.

Materials

Vary according to the activity.

Method

Allow women to come up with their own ideas of things to do – sharing skills and knowledge about our health traditions, and ways of doing things, for example:

- herbal and bush remedies

- teaching ourselves massage techniques

- music (listening to tapes and records or performing and sharing their own talents)

- telling our own stories

- dancing or singing

- celebrating festivals and cultural events

- self-defence, yoga and other physical activities.

These are all health-enhancing activities and allow women to express themselves, their individuality and culture in ways of their choosing.

17C Y'a ba'an b' y'a n'a! (You're born but you're not from)

EXERCISE

Purpose

- To share sayings, quotations, proverbs, wisdom and worldly advice women use or have had passed down to them.

- To assess their value in inspiring black women's lives and promoting their health and identity.

Suitable for

Any stage in a group's life.

Materials

Large sheets of paper (lining paper is cheap). Marker pens, blu-tac, coloured stickers.

Method

1   Lay out the paper where all group members can see it and write on it comfortably. (A large central table is ideal to work on – the floor can pose difficulties for women who are less mobile.)

2   Start with an example of a saying that you have grown up with or come across. (It might be from a relative or friend, school-books, television, and so on.) Write it down on the paper, then get women to write down their own sayings. For example:

- You can't build happiness on other people's unhappiness.

- There is no loss without pain and conflict. All loss can lead to growth.

- There is only one race: the human race.

If women wish, encourage them to discuss their sayings before writing them down.

3   When you have enough (or the group has run out of ideas), go through the sayings one by one. Get the group to put each into one of three categories:

- inspiring (moves us forward)
- just describes reality
- non-inspiring (holds us back)

You could use coloured stickers to mark the differences.

Discussion
If appropriate, facilitate a group discussion on where these sayings come from, how useful they are, and the impact they can have on women's health and well-being.

17D Working on ourselves

E X E R C I S E

Purpose
To promote women's well-being by encouraging them to look within themselves for the qualities they admire in other people.

Suitable for
Early on in a group's life.

Materials
Large pieces of paper, pens.

Method
1   Divide the group into threes.

2   Each woman should take a piece of paper, and think about someone they feel positive about, admire and respect. They should then write down that person's positive qualities.

3   In threes, each woman should now describe her chosen individual to the others. What qualities do these people have in common? Get women to write these on another piece of paper.

4   In the main group, ask women to identify the qualities which came up most strongly or frequently in the small groups.

5   Ask each woman to choose one of these qualities for herself.

Each group member should then say what she has done or will do to demonstrate that she possesses that quality.

Discussion

If appropriate, facilitate a group discussion about the difficulties some black women have in identifying their own positive qualities. You might also want to look at the value and use of role models for black women.

17E Identifying and creating positive images for ourselves

EXERCISE

Purpose

To consider the lack of positive images in black women's lives, and the potential effect of this on their own and their children's self-esteem.

Suitable for

Any stage in a group's life.

Materials

As agreed by group members.

Method

In the absence of sufficient positive images of black women, you might want to focus on activities to create some. Encourage women to discuss these issues for themselves. They could share examples of good resource materials they have come across and look at ways of making them widely known to others. See also the suggestions for activities in exercise 17B.

Discussion

Raise the following points with the group.

- Why is it important for us to have positive images of our community or ourselves as black women?

- What do we mean by positive images? How do positive images – pictures, role models, and so on – affect our self-esteem?

- How can we set about creating positive images if we don't have them already
  - for ourselves?
  - for our children?

Activities

1   An example of creating a positive image for a young child that can be shared in a group is a 'baby frieze' made up of photos or drawings of family members on card, covered in cellophane and fixed as a surround in the baby's pram or room.

2   You could consider making a video about the group and some of its health experiences (if you have access to these resources and can develop your confidence to do this).

3   Consider making various kinds of displays or posters from good photographs of group members, their children and aspects of their lives. There is a particular need for this since black women are often not represented at all in resource materials.

Resources

Planning and facilitating

Bedford, J and Pepper, L J. *Women together: A health education training handbook for ourselves and others.* HEA 1992.

Clarke, D and Underwood, J. *Assertion training.* National Extension College 1988.

Community Education Training Group. *Training and how to enjoy it.* CETG 1989.

Dison, H and Gordon, P. *Working with uncertainty: a handbook for those involved in training on HIV and AIDS.* Family Planning Association 1990.

Fulfilment, J F. *Working more creatively with groups.* Routledge 1991.

Kazowski, S and Land, P. *In our experience.* Women's Press 1988.

Pattenson, L and Burns, J. *Women, assertiveness and health.* HEA 1990.

Sapin, K and Watters, G. *Learning from each other.* William Temple Foundation 1990.

Slavin, H (ed). *Organising health events for women.* HEA 1991.

Szirom, T and Dyson, S. *Greater expectations: a source book for working with girls and young women.* Learning Development Aids 1986.

For all women's groups

Assertiveness

Training packs

Community Education Training Unit. *Assertion and how to train ourselves.* CETU 1990. Available from: CETU, Trinity Royd Cottage, Blackwall, Halifax HX1 3AG. Tel: 0422 357394.

Holland, S and Ward, C. *Assertiveness: a practical approach.* Winslow Press 1990.

McBride, P. *The positive approach: assertiveness resource pack.* Available from: Learning Development Aids, Abbeygate House, East Road, Cambridge CB1 1DB. Tel: 0223 357744.

People First. *Assertiveness package: assertiveness for self-advocacy and self-help groups.* Available from: People First, Instrument House, 207–215 Kings Cross Road, London WC1 9DB. Tel: 071 713 6400.

Richardson, C, Alcoe, J (ed). *Negotiating assertively: a training and self-study package to develop assertive negotiating skills.* Pavilion 1990. Available from: Pavilion Publishing, 8 St George's Place, Brighton BN1 4GB. Tel: 0273 623222.

Strathclyde Regional Council's Women's Unit. *Assertiveness pack for girls and young women.* Available from: Strathclyde Regional Council's Women's Unit, Chief Executive's Dept, 20 India Street, Glasgow G2 4PF. Tel: 041 227 2586/3353.

Townend, A. *Assertion training: a handbook for those involved in training.* Family Planning Association 1991.

Whitehead, C. *So, what is assertiveness? Assertiveness training resource pack.* Daniels Publishing 1992.

Books

Alberti, R. *Your perfect right: a guide to assertive living.* Impact Publishers (US) 1983.

Back, Ken and Kate. *Assertiveness at work.* McGraw Hill 1990.

Bloom, L, Coburn, K, and Pearlman, J. *The new assertive woman.* Laurel Dell (US) 1980.

Cox, G and Dainow, S. *Making the most of yourself.* Sheldon Press 1985.

Dickson, A. *A woman in your own right: assertiveness and you.* Quartet 1982.

Fensterheim, H and Baer, J. *Don't say yes when you want to say no.* Warner 1993.

Hare, B. *Be assertive.* Optima 1988.

Lindenfield, G. *Assert yourself: a self-help assertiveness programme for men and women.* Thorsons 1987.

Lindenfield, G. *Super confidence. Woman's guide to getting what you want out of life.* Thorsons 1992.

Phelps, S and Austin, N. *Assertive woman.* Arlington Books 1988.

Rees, S and Roderick, S. *Assertion training: how to be who you really are.* Routledge 1991.

Steinem, G. *Revolution from within*. Bloomsbury 1992.

Walmsley, C. *Assertiveness, the right to be you*. BBC Books 1991.

Videos

Birmingham Girl Zone Productions. *It's what I want*. 1990. 26 minute video concerning equal opportunities and gender issues. Distributed by: Carola Klein, Girl Zone Productions, 57 Featherstone Road, Birmingham B14 6BD. Tel: 021 443 2131.

Central TV. *A change for the better*. 1986. 30 minute video on the menopause. Available from: Video Resources Centre, Central TV, Central House, Broad Street, Birmingham B1 2JP. Tel: 021 643 9898.

Channel Four TV. *Assert yourself*. 1987. 4 × 40 minute programmes dealing with various aspects of assertiveness.

Concord Video and Film Council. *Toward intimacy*. 62 minute video in which four women with disabilities relate their personal experiences and raise important issues including sexuality and self esteem. Available from: CVFC, 201 Felixstowe Road, Ipswich IP3 9BJ. Tel: 0473 726012/715754.

Edinburgh Film Workshop for Lothian Women and Stress Group. *Stress*. 10 minute video suggests ways of coping with stress in everyday life. Available from: Edinburgh Film Workshop Trust, 29 Albany Street, Edinburgh EH1 3QN. Tel: 031 557 5242.

Franciscan Communications. *Surviving anger: yours and others*. 1989. 32 minute video which discusses the different causes of anger and its various guises. Available from: CTVC, Hillside Studios, Merryhill Road, Bushey, Herts WD2 1DR. Tel: 081 950 4426.

Health Media. *Sex, girls and kiss curls*. 1990. 14 minute video: five women with learning difficulties discuss sex, safer sex, relationships and romance. Available from: Health Media, Health Promotion Unit, Dept of Health New South Wales, Pallister, St Vincents Road, Greenwich, NSW. Tel: 010 612 439 4288.

Leeds Animation Workshop. *All stressed up*. 1993. Looks at the causes and effects of workplace stress, particularly concerning women, and explores the myths that surround it. Available from: LAW. Tel: 0532 484997.

Leeds Vera Productions. *I want to be an astronaut*. 1992. 14 minute video with sketches, street interviews and discussion about freedom of choice, self expression and equal opportunities. Available from: Vera Productions, 30–38 Dock Street, Leeds LS10 1JF. Tel: 0532 428646.

London Borough of Hammersmith and Fulham. *Self defence? Common sense!* 1992. 30 minute video: older women deal positively with self defence. Available from: Pavilion Publishing, 8 St George's Place, Brighton BN1 4GB. Tel: 0273 623222.

Newcastle-upon-Tyne Girls Video Project. *You can say no.* 1987. 40 minute video showing positive images of women saying no in different situations from sexual harassment to sexual abuse and rape. Available from: Albany Video Distribution, Battersea Studios, Television Centre, Thackeray Road, London SW8 3TW. Tel: 071 498 6811.

Health

Packs

Heather, B. *Sharing: a handbook for those involved in training in personal relationships and sexuality.* Family Planning Association 1984.

McCarthy, M and Thompson, D. *Sex and the three Rs: rights, responsibilities and risks.* Pavilion 1992.

Pearson, V. *Women and power: gaining back control.* Pavilion 1992.

Books

Aggleton, P et al. *AIDS: working with young people.* AVERT 1990. Available from: AVERT, 11 Denne Parade, Horsham RH2 1JD. Tel: 0403 210202.

Barbach, LG. *For yourself: the fulfilment of female sexuality.* Doubleday 1975.

Barbach, LG. *For each other: sharing sexual intimacy.* Doubleday 1984.

Boston Women's Health Collective. *Ourselves growing older: women ageing with knowledge and power.* Fontana 1990.

Dickson, A. *The mirror within: a new look at sexuality.* Quartet Books 1980.

Dison, H. *Chance to choose: sexuality and relationships education for people with learning difficulties.* Learning Development Aids 1992.

Dixon, H and Mullinar, G. *Taught not caught: strategies for sex education.* Learning Development Aids 1989.

Dowling, S. *Health for a change: provision of preventative healthcare in pregnancy and early childhood.* Child Poverty Action Group 1984.

Greer, G. *The change: women, ageing, and the menopause.* Hamish Hamilton 1991.

Hayman, S. *The well woman handbook: a guide for women throughout their lives*. Penguin 1989.

Hemmings, S. *A wealth of experience: the lives of older women*. Pandora 1985.

Hemmings, S (ed). *True to life: writings by young women*. Sheba 1986.

Hepburn, C and Gutierez, B. *Alive and well: lesbian health guide*. Crossing Press (US) 1989.

Kitzinger, S. *Woman's experience of sex*. Penguin 1985.

Mariasy, J and Thomas, L. *Triple jeopardy: women and AIDS*. Panos Publications 1990.

Markham, U. *Women under pressure: a practical guide for today's woman*. Element Books 1990.

Mosse J and Heaton, J. *The fertility and contraception book*. Faber & Faber 1990.

O'Sullivan, S and Parmar, P. *Lesbians talk (safer) sex*. Scarlet Press 1992.

Phillips, A & Rakusen, G. *The new our bodies ourselves: a health book by and for women*. Penguin 1989.

Reitz, R. *Menopause: a positive approach*. Harvester Press 1979.

Rowe, D. *Choosing not losing: the experience of depression*. Fontana 1988.

Tidyman, M and Furedi, A. *Women's health guide*. HEA (forthcoming).

Workers' Education Association. *Every woman's health: information and resources for group discussion*. Health Education Authority 1993.

For black women's groups

General resources

Age Concern, Lewisham. *Fact: you are never too old to enjoy sex.* 1993. Poster for older people from black and minority ethnic groups. Available from: Age Concern Lewisham, 20 Brown Hill Road, Catford, London SE6 2EN. Tel: 081 695 6000 ext. 3352.

Bolton Centre for Health Promotion. *Health information for women* – periods, thrush, cystitis, breast care, family planning, cervical smear testing, safer sex and HIV (English, Gujarati and

Urdu). 1992. Available from: Bolton Centre for Health Promotion, Bolton Health Authority, 3 Chorley New Road, Bolton BL1 4QR. Tel: 0204 32089.

Bolton Centre for Health Promotion. *Menopause: a time to look forward* (English, Gujarati and Urdu). 1992.

Bryan, B, Dadzie, S, and Scafe, S. *The heart of the race: black women's lives in Britain*. Virago 1985.

Cobham, M and Collins, R. *Watchers and seekers: poetry by black women*. The Women's Press 1987.

D-Ashur, S. *Silent tears*. London Black Women's Health Action Project 1989. Booklet to accompany the video (see page 220).

Grewal, S et al. *Charting the journey: writings by black and third world women*. Sheba 1988.

Karmi, G (ed). *The ethnic health bibliography*. N E and N W Thames Regional Health Authorities 1993.

Kings Healthcare. *Listen my sister . . . putting AIDS into context*. Pack – information on women's health, HIV and AIDS and race. 1992. Available from: Kings Healthcare, 94–104 Denmark Hill, London SE5 8RX. Tel: 071 738 6181.

London Race and Housing Research Unit. *The hidden struggle*. LRHU 1989. Statutory and voluntary responses to violence against black women in the home.

Mares, P, Henley, A, and Baxter, C. *Health care in multiracial Britain*. National Extension College 1985. Illustrated handbook which explores the key issues included in developing health services to meet the needs of a multiracial population. Available from: NEC, 18 Brookland Avenue, Cambridge CB2 2HN. Tel: 0223 316644.

McNeill, P et al. *Through the break: women in personal struggle*. Sheba Feminist Publishers 1987.

Positively Women. *African women's health issues*. Positively Women 1992. Information leaflet about HIV and AIDS. Available from: Positively Women, 5 Sebastian Street, London EC1V 0HE. Tel: 071 490 5501.

Smyke, P. *Women and health*. ZED Books 1992.

Torkington, N P K. *Black health: a political issue*. Health and Race Project 1991.

Wilson, A. *Finding a voice: Asian women in Britain*. Virago 1978.

White, E C. *Chain, chain, change: for black women dealing with physical and emotional abuse*. Seal Press 1986.

White, E C (ed). *Black women's health book: speaking for ourselves*. Seal Press 1990.

Videos

Asian Community Arts. *Great expectations*. 1992. 15 minute video: Asian youth workers talk about the need for specialist services for young Asians, particularly young women. Available from: Black Issues in Community Arts, Hyde Youth and Community Centre, Lower Bennett Street, Hyde SK14 1PP.

Azad Productions. *A fearful silence*. 1985. 52 minute video examines how domestic violence affects three Asian women. Available from: Albany Video Distribution, Battersea Studios, Television Centre, Thackeray Road, London SW8 3TW. Tel: 071 498 6811.

Berkshire Education Department Resources Unit. *In their own words*. 1989. 59 minute video: Asian women present their views on life, work and experiences. Available from: Dramatic Distribution, 79 London Street, Reading RG1 4QA. Tel: 0734 394170.

Department of Health. *Your right to health*. 28 minute video: to encourage the use of the NHS and familiarise the Chinese community with hospital and GP services (Cantonese). Available from: CFL Vision, PO Box 35, Wetherby, W Yorks LS23 7EX. Tel: 0937 541010.

London Black Women's Health Action Project. *Silent tears*: an educational programme about female circumcision. 1990. 20 minute video providing information to counteract ignorance and raise awareness about the issues surrounding female genital mutilation. Available from: London Black Women's Health Action Project, Neighbourhood Building, 1 Cornwall Avenue, London E2 0HW. Tel: 081 980 3503.

London Chinese Health Resource Centre. *The breast self-examination and the gynaecological examination*. 1990. 20 minute video for Chinese women (Cantonese). Available from: Healthcare Productions Ltd, 2 Stucley Place, Camden Lock, London NW1 8NS. Tel: 071 267 8757.

N Films. *Hysterectomy*. 1991. 23 minute video for Asian women who may have had or be about to have a hysterectomy (English, Bengali, Hindi, Punjabi, Urdu). Available from: N Films, 78 Holyhead Road, Handsworth, Birmingham B21 0LH. Tel: 021 507 0341.

Scan Video Productions. *I see from here*. 1988. 14 minute video in which a group of women talk about what it is like to be a young Asian person living in Britain. Available from Albany Video Distribution, Battersea Studios, Television Centre, Thackeray Road, London SW8 3TW. Tel: 071 498 6811.

Shanti Asian Women and Stress Project. *Shanti stress pack*. 1991. 45 minute video and 60 minute audio cassette: skills and information for Asian women to manage stress (English,

Bengali, Urdu). Available from: Shanti Asian Women and Stress Project, Health Promotion Services, Coventry Health Authority, Coventry and Warwickshire Hospital, Stoney Stanton Road, Coventry CV1 4FH. Tel: 0203 844092.